Don't Let The Bastards Grind You Down

by Georgia W.

Cover Design by Steve Dickenson
Book Design/Back Cover by Nikki Ward, Morrison Alley Design
Author Illustration by Steve Kiene

First Printing 2009
ISBN 978-0-9817088-0-5
Library of Congress Control Number: 2008910250

For Eric and Christine W.

Contents

Acknowledgements

My love and appreciation to Matt for encouraging me to write this book, for loving me when I'm crazy, and for always being in my corner. Thank you for your editing skills and patience – especially with my addiction to semi-colons (I'm getting help!)

Thank you to Sam, the best sister in the world. I'm extremely grateful for you and so very proud. Also, a big thank you to Mum for your support, and for telling me to 'Keep up the good work, Chuck.' And, of course, I cannot express the gratitude I feel towards my friends, Tom C., Jeff M. and Mark S., for always being there, no matter what.

And a very special thank you to all the people in recovery who told me to "keep coming back" – if you hadn't I might not be here today.

About This Book

"Don't let the bastards grind you down" was a phrase my dad used all the time; he even wrote it on birthday and holiday cards before he signed his name. Back then, I didn't realize it was a well-known saying that had been around for years. I just figured that, for whatever reason, my dad just thought people were bastards.

One of the most notable people to use the expression was an American, General "Vinegar Joe" Stilwell, who adopted it during the Second World War in order to rally his troops against the enemy. Although my dad was never a soldier and didn't fight in any war, he certainly had his share of demons to battle. His number one enemy was "King Alcohol." Everything—and everyone—took a backseat to his drinking. And unfortunately, even though he tried at times, this was a fight my dad would never win.

Dad never did get sober, dying suddenly at age sixty. He just dropped dead one day in the middle of the street. He didn't have any money in his pocket, or any form of identification. In fact, the only thing the coroner passed along to us (once he'd been able to locate our family) was a set of keys and an unopened bottle of Scotch. The irony of this was not lost on my sister and me as we unceremoniously opened the bottle. We hated Scotch, but it was the right thing to do—Dad would have wanted it that way. At least, that's what our alcoholic minds told us.

You see, my dad was an alcoholic, my sister is an alcoholic, and I'm an alcoholic. And that's just my immediate family, the tip of the proverbial iceberg. We are part of a lineage that has an unfortunate legacy of abusing booze and drugs. Our family tree on both sides is littered with alcoholics and addicts. In other words, we produce addicts like the Kennedy clan produces politicians.

It might not have been a surprise that my father had a problem, and maybe trouble was always in the cards for my sister and me. But while Dad may have been an alcoholic and a less than perfect father, he was a good, decent man, and his attitude and sense of humor have helped me to make it through my own recovery. I have come to realize that "Don't let the bastards grind you down" was the best he could do in the way of a father-daughter talk. And I guess it must have resonated with me, because I often found myself saying it as a kind of mantra in my early recovery. It seemed then as if I'd also inherited Dad's distaste for people, mainly because they were always trying to piss on my parade.

Why were people always on my case? Well, by the age of thirty-six I had become a pretty hopeless alcoholic myself by most people's standards. I'd been trying to get sober for four years. Sure, I could stop drinking, but I couldn't *stay stopped*. I had spent the last few years in a vicious cycle: two to three months sober, followed by a bout of drinking, then intense guilt, remorse, and hopelessness before the whole thing would start over again. My life was a nightmare. The way I saw it, I had two options: get sober for good, or kill myself. After some consideration, I came to the conclusion that if I succeeded in committing suicide, I'd most likely go to a place not unlike hell. And in my particular version of hell there would be *no booze,* which was an inconceivable thought. Or, if by some karmic fluke, I ended up in a place like heaven, then there would *definitely be no booze*, so I was out of luck either way.

As I think about that now, I realize how unbelievably crazy it sounds, but at the time the absence of alcohol in both of those after-life scenarios really was the only reason I could come up with to not kill myself. Alcohol owned me, and I couldn't imagine how I'd keep living with it or ever manage to get through the day without it. I was even trying to plan my afterlife around it, and worst of all, it never even entered my head that such thinking might be a little odd.

After years of failing miserably, I was at a complete loss and wanted more than anything to find a sense of direction and purpose. So, after yet another relapse, I decided to try recovery again. I had heard that the best way to learn about *real* recovery was from someone who'd been through it, so I decided to do some research, specifically looking for books written by other alcoholics or addicts. What I found were a lot of memoirs detailing people's sobriety stories along with the obvious Twelve-Step program guides. There were also plenty of books written by people with important-sounding letters and titles after their names, and they all seemed very knowledgeable and profound—the only problem was, I couldn't concentrate long enough to read them. I needed something short and easy to read, something a bit simpler. After all, I was new in recovery; my head was in a daze and I had the attention span of a gnat.

Amazingly enough, and through a lot of trial and error (as you read on, you'll see what I mean), I managed to stay sober for longer than my customary two to three months. After some time had passed, I decided to write about what I had learned from my failure and success. I wanted to write that simple guide I had searched for and hadn't been able to find when I'd started my recovery.

The goal of this book is to highlight some things that all of us should know *after* we've come to the conclusion that we have an alcohol or drug problem and have decided to try recovery. If you are still on the fence and are unsure if you have a problem, then you may need further proof until it becomes clear to you. However, if alcohol or drugs have become enough of an issue in your life that you are taking a look at this book, then chances are, you could use some help.

There are a hundred reasons why you may want to quit, but the most important reason is that *you're* ready. If you are doing this for someone else—a spouse, family member, employer, or even the courts—know that a time will come when you'll have to decide if you want sobriety for yourself, or if you're just going through the motions to please someone else. Usually, that moment is where the rubber really meets the road, when you'll either use again or you won't.

If you're ready to move on to a life without drinking or drugs, I invite you to read on. My aim was to write a book that *any* alcoholic or addict who is brand new to recovery or trying recovery again could easily understand. This journey isn't going to be easy, but I promise you it will be worth it in the end. It's irrelevant how you got to this point in your life—the important part is that you *did*, and everything else will fall into place if you are willing to follow the advice of people who have been there before. The bad news is that too many alcoholics and addicts die before they get to the point you are at right now. But there is good news: *Anybody* can get clean and sober. I'm living proof—what experts call a chronic alcoholic—and if I can do it, there's no reason why you can't either.

Best of all, you don't have to do it all by yourself. There are dozens of different recovery programs out there, and lots of people who want to help, but it all has to start with you. By openly listening and learning about the disease of addiction and by choosing to pick up this book instead of a drink or a drug, you're taking a step in the right direction. Even if it feels as though you can't concentrate long enough to read just a few pages at a time, it's a start.

I hope all of the tools and advice in these pages will help you on your journey. The first half of the book concentrates on what to expect in early recovery, while the remainder is about actually having a *life* in recovery, covering Twelve-Step programs, what's involved, and my experience with them.

There will be differences between my story and yours, but you will probably see lots of similarities, too. With that in mind, please take what you can use and leave what you can't. Good luck!

#1. The First 30 Days

there's a good reason why people say the first thirty days are the hardest part of recovery—because they are. It's not so much that we are "in recovery" as hanging on for dear life. During this first stretch, the obsession to use can feel like it will never leave us. In fact, I felt as though nothing short of a miracle could make it go away. This is by far the toughest part, and it will take all of your determination and effort just to make it through. The good news, however, is that when you *do* make it through the first month, you'll come out the other side feeling better than you have in a very long time.

I realize this information isn't actually that helpful when you're in your first month, because it feels like an eternity. In fact, if you concentrate on trying to make it through an entire thirty days, you're probably going to feel overwhelmed. The key is to think small and keep your head within each twenty-four hour period. Sometimes even this might seem like too much. If the idea of getting through a day feels like a lot, then try managing hourly increments.

The beginning is hard; there's no question about it, but if I did it, you can too. During my first month, I felt like I was coming undone at a nearly constant pace. Sometimes I felt unable to speak and I wanted to be alone; then at other times I wanted to scream and cry, randomly punch people, crawl out of my skin, or jump off a building at any given moment—mainly because the idea of being sober seemed like such an insurmountable task. If you find yourself feeling like that, it might help to look at it this way: As addicts, we've abused the hell out of ourselves, often for months or years. Now our bodies are in shock, our minds are confused and disoriented, and we generally loathe everything and everybody, including ourselves. We didn't get sick overnight, and we certainly won't get well overnight, either. But this will pass and things will get better, if you can just hang in there for another twenty-four hours.

It's not unusual for the struggle to be the hardest during the first week after your last drink or drug. You'll likely experience intense cravings, as well as the withdrawal effects that come with removing the addictive substance from your body. That's why medical detox can be so helpful in the beginning. Those seven days or so are a very important time, as far as your physical well-being is concerned. Your body, used to a constant flow of poison, may feel jolted. You will probably suffer from symptoms like headaches, vomiting, and sweats. It's not unusual for alcoholics to experience seizures when we stop drinking abruptly. Managing these symptoms can be a dangerous part of your recovery. If you find that in the past you have had severe nausea or tremors, or if you've generally had a very difficult time sobering up or coming down from drugs, you might want to consider seeking professional help at your local hospital or clinic for at least the first one to five days. If this is not an option for you, try to make sure you have someone who can check on you daily or even stay with you through the first three days.

After seven days, you might start to feel a gradual difference, although most new people in recovery tend to be in a bit of a fog for the first few weeks. Expect that your mind will be cloudy and your body will feel weak. It will probably still be difficult to focus for long periods of time. When I was a few months clean, I tried to recall what I'd done during the first thirty days, and I couldn't remember much.

This is the time when you need to just stick with your basic survival needs: sleeping, eating, and working (if you still have a job). Bathing now and again might be a good idea, too. And as trivial as it may sound, developing a regular sleep routine and trying to eat three meals a day are very important. Rest and nutrition can do wonders to help your body and mind recover more quickly, especially if you've been going without either or both for a long time.

In the beginning, coffee and cigarettes tend to be the staple of most recovery diets. I certainly took in my share of caffeine and nicotine during my first few months, and I won't try to talk you out of them if you're in the habit. Obviously, neither one is very good for you; nor is anything done in excess. But, that being said, this book isn't about quitting smoking or drinking coffee, so I wouldn't worry too much about it. Getting through the first month is a huge accomplishment. If doing that takes a gallon of coffee a day and one too many cigarettes, then that's what it takes. You probably won't harm yourself a tenth as much as you would have if you were drinking or using, and besides, you can always look at quitting other things later, if you choose to (like I did).

Once the "brain fog" starts to lift, we're able to start thinking a little more clearly, retaining information better. At this point, you can start to make some progress against your addiction if you can stay focused and keep your thoughts where they need to be. A great way to stay on track is using your mornings effectively to set the tone for the rest of the day. For me, the most powerful tool was reading. There are some great books with readings and meditations in them specifically for people in recovery (see the list of suggested reading in the back of the book). Studying a few of them after you wake up in the morning to get focused, settle your mind, and relax your body can help you gear up for the day ahead. It only takes a few minutes, and it could make all the difference.

Once you've had a few quiet moments to think, try to make an effort to eat something for breakfast, even if it's just a cereal bar and a cup of coffee or juice. By the same token, exercise might be the last thing on your mind, but introducing just a little into your routine, even just a short walk, will help with your appetite and sleeping. Getting out of your home or job and going for a ten minute walk really helps clear the head and re-energize the body, as long as you avoid the street where the liquor store or the dealer is.

If you are in a Twelve-Step program, you should try to attend at least one meeting a day for the first ninety days of your recovery. If you have a hard time finding a free hour or two, it might help to remember the hours and days that were wasted on drinking and using. Couldn't you put some of that same effort into your recovery? If you truly can't make it, or lack transportation, be aware that some programs offer online meetings and clean and sober chat rooms. If you do not have a computer or Internet at home, your local library should have access.

The point is to make your recovery program, whatever it might entail, a part of your daily routine. If you do not want to try a Twelve-Step program, you could use the time to do some research online for other recovery options that you might want to consider (see Chapter 44, "The Agnostic and Atheist").

Recovery is like a full-time job, and we need to stay on top of it in order to succeed. If we put the work in, we'll reap the rewards. But, just like our real jobs, it can't be all work and no play. It's very important to find the right balance and know our limitations. Sometimes it's okay that the only thing on our "To Do" list for the day is *"Don't drink or drug."*

From time to time, after a really intense or exhausting day, we might be susceptible to "emotional hangovers." In the same way we used to get hangovers when we'd go overboard with booze or drugs, leaving our bodies suffering, emotional hangovers occur when we've been pushed to the limit mentally, causing us to suffer psychologically. When you're not used to it, being present and facing reality on a daily basis can be very demanding. At times we're so drained from "feeling too much" that we lose the ability to feel *anything*. You'll know you've reached this point when you feel overwhelmed and want to rest. The best way to deal with it? If your schedule allows, simply *rest* for a day and don't beat yourself up over it. If you can't take a day off, try taking a short nap or a walk during lunch. You'll be surprised how much these small things can revitalize the mind and body.

No matter where you are in your first month, concentrate on the day or hour that you're in. Thinking through small bits of time takes the pressure off, keeps your sobriety from becoming too overwhelming, and keeps you in the here and now. Is it really going to matter, in the grand scheme of things, if you don't make your bed for once? How does that compare to the accomplishment of managing to stay clean and sober for another day? Whether we're in recovery or not, all any of us have is *today*. If we get ahead of ourselves and think about tomorrow's problems, we're wasting our energy on the future and ignoring the present.

Keep your day simple, don't try to take on the world, and don't worry, the bed will still need making tomorrow.

#2. The Disease

an addiction is a dependence, either on a *substance*, like alcohol or drugs, or a *behavior*, like gambling or sex. You've probably realized that by now, even if you never thought of your problem in those terms. What you might not know, however, is that your addiction is in fact a disease. This concept came as quite a surprise to me, as it seems to for most people in recovery.

In fact, I remember exactly when I was first presented with this idea. It happened during one of my attempts at sobriety, when I was sitting in a treatment center meeting with a dozen or so other hapless and hopeless souls. At that moment, the counselor said those magic words: *"Addiction is a disease*. You can't help it; you were born this way."* I felt like I'd won the lottery! Finally, someone had said it out loud: It's a disease. All my bad behavior wasn't my fault—the disease made me do it! This was more than music to my ears; it was like getting a free pass on everything that had gone wrong with my life.

Obviously, I still had a lot to learn. While I was busy blaming all of my problems on something else and generally avoiding accountability for anything, what little I had left kept on crumbling around me. Still, I carried on with this notion that my disease was to blame for all my troubles until one day I realized I'd lost everything that mattered in my life. I found myself jobless, broke, divorced without custody of my son, and sleeping on a friend's couch. It finally dawned on me that I was responsible for the situation in which I found myself. Booze didn't do this—I did. Alcohol wasn't helping, but I was the one who kept drinking it even though I knew that I had a disease, a disease that left me unable to stop using once I'd started. The ball was in my court. I was aware of my condition, and I had to do everything in my power to not put alcohol in my system in the first place. I came to realize the truth: I have a disease, not an excuse, and it is solely my responsibility to treat it.

As addicts, one of the best things we can do, for ourselves and others, is to face up to our disease and realize it for what it is. On the one hand, it's a legitimate medical problem, and we have to accept that our biology deserves some of the blame. On the other side of the coin, though, we're left with an obligation to take that information and get help. Having an addiction isn't an excuse to use, anymore than having diabetes is an excuse to pass out from low blood sugar while driving on the highway. Diseases need to be treated, not ignored.

Also, realize that many people will not be as sympathetic to your condition as you'd like. When it comes to treating addiction as a medical phenomenon, there are a lot of skeptics out there. There are going to be people in your life who think you have a problem because you are weak, lack willpower, or have little moral fiber. Non-addicts, or "normal people," as I will refer to them throughout this book, have a hard time understanding our addiction, much less why we do the things we do. For that reason, we tend to incite frustration and impatience in them. You've probably heard the question "Why can't you just stop?" a hundred times, as I certainly did.

However, most experts believe that we alcoholics and addicts are born this way. In other words, our disease is like a time bomb, lying dormant in our genes until we light the fuse by taking that first drink or drug. Once we do, we set off a craving in our bodies that is not present in normal people. We're just wired differently, and that keeps us from stopping when we should, as normal people do.

I have a vivid recollection of my first "drunk" because I had a moment of clarity that seemed very out of the ordinary for a twelve-year-old. My sister and I had taken brandy from a friend's parent's house. We snuck away to have a try, and when I took that first drink, the switch flipped. I felt its warmth spread into my stomach, through my chest, my head, and the rest of my body. I immediately wanted *more*, and after a few further sips, I was overcome with a sensation of being giddy, coupled with a feeling of calm and peace. That's when I knew. I had a sense of foreboding (okay, I didn't know what foreboding was at twelve, but I felt very weird, nonetheless) and I knew, without a shadow of a doubt, that I was in deep shit. I actually said out loud, to no one in particular, "I'm going to have a problem with this my whole life; I'm going to be just like my dad."

When I look back at that moment, I think the fact that I said "my whole life" was actually a bit profound. I was only twelve, and my scope of thinking didn't usually go that far. For the most part, it was all about what cartoons I was going to watch that afternoon, yet I just knew this would be with me for life. You'd think this epiphany would have stopped me from ever picking up a bottle again, but I'd just lit the fuse to the time bomb.

Still, it would be many years until I imploded, although the timeline seems to be a bit different for each person. Sometimes the disease takes hold in just a few months; other times we go along for years, slipping away bit by bit. Regardless of the schedule, though, the end is always the same—things get progressively worse until we come to a point where we are physically unable to stop. This is where the insanity of the addiction begins: We want to stop, but we can't. Or, we continually try to control how much we use, promising ourselves "just one more," even though we know it never ends up that way. More often than not, we find ourselves waking up from a blackout, sometimes a day or a week later, and wondering how we got there. The "lucky ones" manage to stay on their feet, weaving through each day in an altered state by maintaining a certain level of booze or drugs in their system in order to function at an acceptable level, or one that seems acceptable to them but probably not to everyone else. The harsh reality is that once we reach this point of no return in our drinking or using careers, we can never go back to a couple of drinks in the evening or recreational drug use on the weekends. We will never regain control.

With the knowledge that our addiction is an illness we can't control, we can understand how best to fight it, and why we need to do so. Respect the power of your problem, but don't hide behind it. By acknowledging that we have a disease, we also have to acknowledge our own responsibility to treat it.

Alcoholism was recognized by the American Medical Association as an illness in 1957. Since then, addiction has been validated as a medical condition for both alcoholism and drug addiction by professional associations worldwide, including the British Medical Association.

#3. Dry Drunk

the term "dry drunk" is a derogatory name for people who are no longer physically drinking or using, even though their personalities, behaviors, and attitudes are the same as when they were. In other words, they're bad-tempered, antisocial, and often depressed. They exhibit the same traits they did while using, such as dishonesty, cheating, and selfishness, to name just a few. Basically, nothing has changed except they're no longer putting their drug of choice into their bloodstreams. They do not have a recovery program in place, so while they might be clean and sober, they are also utterly miserable and barely hanging on.

I experienced the feeling of being a dry drunk a number of times when I tried to quit on my own. It was torture. Even though I was no longer using, I was preoccupied with it constantly. Every day was the same. I would wake up with a knot in my stomach as the realization, "Oh no, I can't drink today," dawned on me, which would be followed by an entire day spent obsessively thinking about how *not* to drink, or what would happen if I did. At the end of it all, I'd go to bed as early as possible to get the day over with and put a stop to the mental merry-go-round. Finally, after months of feeling like shit, I would inevitably cave in and seek relief in my drug of choice.

Even though I wasn't using, alcohol still controlled my mind. I was thinking about it constantly, and I decided that if this was what sobriety meant, then I didn't want it. I wasn't going to spend my life in a state of constant obsession and misery, craving what I couldn't have; it was better just to use again and hope I'd die sooner rather than later. The problem with that idea is, this disease *will* kill us, but we never know exactly *when*. We could be looking at years of abusing ourselves, living in a half-dead state, until we actually succumb to a very painful death. Deciding to give up isn't such an easy way out after all.

I went through my time as a dry drunk because I tried to do things on my own. I learned that for me, like most people, willpower just isn't enough. It was a tough lesson, but at least it made me realize I was being naïve by hoping that I could abstain from a substance I was physically addicted to with no defense other than my mind. Living life that way—dreading every morning, being angry, pissed-off, and constantly craving my drug of choice—wasn't going to cut it. It could only lead to relapse, whether it was one week, one month, or one year down the line.

I had no choice but to try something else, so I decided to do the one thing I'd been avoiding for years. I was going to go to a recovery meeting, one of those places where all those 'really fucked-up people' went.

#4. The Real Problem

Just as someone else can't force us to get clean and sober in the first place, we can't be made to believe that we are an alcoholic or an addict, either. We have to self-diagnose. We can tell people what they want to hear, but unless we actually believe it, it doesn't make a blind bit of difference. Before we can successfully treat our disease, we have to fully admit to ourselves that we actually have one to begin with. Sure, doctors might tell us that we have all the signs of alcoholism or addiction, but as of yet, there's no blood test to diagnose it and no magic pill to treat it.

Everybody I knew seemed to think I was an alcoholic, but I spent years inwardly denying it. I didn't want to admit it, because I knew that if I did, it was the end of the road as far as my drinking was concerned, and I wasn't ready to let go of my crutch. It was at the recovery meetings that I really got a sense of what it meant to be an addict. And it was there that I finally got to the point of admitting to *myself* that I was an alcoholic. This was a very big deal to me, worthy of a parade or at least a pat on the back! Shortly after I'd made my breakthrough, though, someone had to go and piss on my parade like they always did. They sat me down and told me something that just had to be absolute crap (mainly because I didn't understand it). They actually had the nerve to tell me that alcohol and drugs were just a symptom of something greater and that, get this, *I was the problem.*

Like I said, when I first heard this statement, I didn't really understand it. All I heard was this nut saying that I was the problem, not the booze, and immediately I went on the defensive. No one was going to blame me for anything! Despite that, he went on to say that I just happened to use my drug of choice as a temporary "bandage" to cover up the real issue, which was me (I didn't like that at all). I wanted to punch him in the face (as was my typical response in early recovery), and I listed countless examples of things that had happened to me, or that I'd done while under the influence, to substantiate my point that I only behaved that way when I used.

The half-wit telling me otherwise suggested I listen to what other people had to say about this idea before I dismissed it. I stopped ranting and raving for long enough to sit in the meetings and listen to the "old timers," people who had been in recovery for a long time. All the while, I felt absolutely convinced that they'd say something to agree with my argument and enable me to say "I told you so" to the half-wit.

After listening and talking more extensively with other addicts and hearing about their experiences in recovery, it seemed that we did have one thing in common: Most of us thought that when we stopped using our drug of choice, our problems would disappear, everything would be perfect, and things could get back to normal. We thought all of our troubles were consequences of our addiction, and every bad thing that happened was a direct result of our using. It seemed only logical that if we took away the cause of our problems, we would no longer have any.

Like the others, I was starting to see that things didn't work that way. I was sure I wasn't a dry drunk anymore, because I was going to recovery meetings, but after two months of attending them, I realized I still didn't feel "normal" at all. Quite the opposite happened. I felt like I was losing my mind, largely because my inner voice wouldn't shut up. I'm not talking about actual voices, telling me the neighbors are aliens and the VW Beetle in their garage was actually a UFO (well, it was silver). I'm talking about the constant stream of thoughts and images that ran through my mind; they were random and obscure but still very real to me. These ideas were both scattered and obsessive. I couldn't stop thinking about the past; the same events replayed again and again. I had so many regrets and so much guilt, not to mention paranoia about the future. What's more, there were all these people that I couldn't stop thinking about. It didn't matter who it was; if someone had hurt me, I couldn't let it go, no matter how minor or how severe the pain they had caused. It didn't matter if it was an old boyfriend who'd beaten me up, or someone who'd stolen my parking spot—they all took up equal space in my head!

From talking with other people in recovery, I learned that this is how our addict brains are. It's the mental part of the disease; we just don't think like normal people. For instance, normal people deal with someone cutting them off in traffic by getting angry for a second, but then they get over it. We react differently. We'll spend a sleepless night staring at the ceiling replaying different scenarios in our minds, kicking ourselves for not doing or saying something to the person who pissed us off.

Most of us (or at least those who admit it), have a constantly running mind and are deluged with obsessive thoughts. I even have a name for mine. I call them "The Hamsters," because it felt like I had a family of them living in my head, constantly running on their wheels, round and round. They never got tired; they never rested, and so they kept my mind going twenty-four hours a day, seven days a week. I was restless, irritable, and totally miserable. The thought of a drink began to sound like a good idea. I just knew I was going insane, and that I was the only one who felt this way, so there was no way I was going to tell anyone what was going on inside my crackpot skull. They'd lock me up and throw away the key!

That went on until I started listening to the other people in the recovery meeting, just like I had been told to. Much to my amazement, I found that I wasn't alone.* There were other people who were just as bat-shit crazy as I was. Not only could they relate to what I was saying, they had hamsters of their own. They might have had a different name for them (I've heard it called "The Committee"), but it all boiled down to the same thing: We all had something in common.

When we stop using our substance of choice, we are only treating the physical symptom of our addiction. We still have the same mind that we always had, and so we need to realize that when the drug is gone, very often our heads go off to the races. Through my own experience, and through talking with other addicts and alcoholics in recovery, I came to the realization that my new friend (the half-wit) was right; alcohol was just a symptom of my condition, and *I was the problem.* For me, recognizing this was just as significant as admitting I was an alcoholic.

We are not alone. According to Substance Abuse and Mental Health Services Administration's 2007 statistics, an estimated 22.3 million Americans – or roughly nine percent of the population over the age of twelve – were classified with substance dependence or abuse.

Citation:

Substance Abuse and Mental Health Services Administration, Office of Applied Studies (2008). *Results from the 2007 National Survey on Drug Use and Health: National Findings* (NSDUH Series H-34, DHHS Publication No. SMA 08-4343). Rockville, MD.

#5. Fighting Our Disease

in war, sometimes even the most fearless of soldiers call for reinforcements, and by conceding their need for help, they may ultimately save their own lives. They know battles are not won single-handedly, and whether we believe it or not, we are also in a fight for our lives.

However, when it comes to asking for help, we alcoholics and addicts tend to be very reluctant. We see it as a sign of weakness, often hoping we can get through it on our own, as though asking for support will make us appear vulnerable or weak. This way of thinking is the mental part of our disease joining forces with our ego, and for most of us, it doesn't end well.

We tend to feel alone and isolated. We might secretly want help, but other people can't read our minds, and so we bottle things up until we come apart, usually in the form of a relapse. We feel as though we're the only ones fighting a battle like this, but nothing could be further from the truth. That's why, in order to fight the battle and win the war, one of the most important things we can do for ourselves is to swallow our false sense of pride. We need to start practicing self-preservation by asking for help, because there really is safety in numbers.

To stave off that isolated feeling, start by developing a list of people who know you are in recovery. Some of them should be in recovery themselves, while others could be family members or friends who want to support you. Keep a list of these people by your phone at home, and programmed into your cell phone. Then comes the hard part: Call them! If you are feeling down or just want to talk with someone, and especially if you want to drink or drug, pick up the phone and use it.

If you have started to go to recovery meetings, speak up. Tell the other attendees you are new and would like to get to know people. You'll be surprised at the how many of them will approach you afterward. In fact, most meetings have a phone list specifically designed for new people to connect with others. It's especially important to speak up if you are having trouble and need help. If you can't share in front of everyone, go up to someone after the meeting and ask if they might be able to talk for a few minutes.

After one of the first recovery meetings I went to, I asked a stranger if I could tag along to another meeting with them that I'd heard them talk about. They agreed without a moment's hesitation. Off we went, and after that meeting was over, I went out for coffee with a group of people I'd only met that night. Later, I realized how out of character it was for me to approach an unfamiliar person like that, but something had made me do it. Maybe it was because my life was on the line, but that stranger has since become one of my closest friends in recovery.

Believe it or not, those already in recovery want to help others who are new. I've heard it compared to the survivor mentality often seen after an accident or natural disaster, in which the people who live to tell the tale seem to develop a special bond. It's only natural, since they can relate to each other on a totally different level than those who haven't experienced the same things.

In order to fight our disease, we have to stick together to help each other. One of the most important things we can do is have a list of reinforcements who won't think twice about coming to our aid and fighting alongside us when the going gets tough.

#6. Some Things You Might Want To Avoid

It's a good idea to avoid making any major changes in your life in early recovery. This suggestion is based on the amount of stress involved in something like marriage, divorce, moving to a new house, switching jobs, or relocating to a new city or town. While it may seem that a fresh start is exactly what's needed, a major upheaval puts a lot of added pressure on you, and that can lead to falling back into old habits.

Sometimes, change can't be avoided. Maybe you or your spouse has a new job that requires relocating, or you've lost your job and you need to look for a new one. If you have no choice, go ahead and do what you have to do, but be sure that you have a safety net in place. Keep phone numbers of sober friends who you can call to talk to, and don't be afraid to use them; you are not alone. Remember, even good change is usually stressful, and if you aren't careful, you could find yourself in trouble.

If you are relocating, do some research on your new town or city. Go online and look for social clubs with sober activities and recovery meetings. New jobs can be tough, especially if you were let go from your previous employer because of your substance problem. If you find yourself in that position, try to reach out to other contacts within your old company. References don't have to come from supervisors, and former fellow employees might be willing to say a few kind words about you.

Relationships might be the biggest stressor of all, particularly if you're ending a marriage or other long-term partnership. That's why, unless there's an immediate danger to you or your recovery, it's recommend that you put off this kind of change. Separating from someone you share your life with can cause a lot of stress that we aren't well-equipped to deal with in early recovery. Furthermore, you and your partner are most likely experiencing a lot of mixed emotions—especially guilt, hurt, and anger—and before the relationship can get better, it usually feels like it's getting worse. That doesn't mean those relationships can't be salvaged and ultimately improved.

A friend of mine in recovery had been married fourteen years when she got sober. By then, her marriage looked like it was down for the count. Both parties decided to stick with it, though, even though they wanted to walk away at times. Now that she's been sober for four years, both partners are grateful they hung in there. In hindsight, they realize that splitting up would have been a decision made when he was still very angry, and she was still very sick. Even though she wasn't still using, she was still dealing with her disease. You'll be surprised how much you can change in that first year, and if you are able to get through it together and find that you still want to end the relationship, then at least you will know that you gave it your best shot. By making the effort, you might just learn that there's hope in the end; you may still love that person for all of their wonderful qualities (and faults), and they may still love you.

Just as it's a good idea not to make hasty decisions regarding ending relationships early in recovery, you really shouldn't start a new relationship, either. Of course, this is easier said than done, and most of us learn the hard way. After looking and feeling like the walking dead for so long, we tend to jump in with both feet if someone is even remotely attracted to us. Suddenly we have a new purpose in life! This works wonders while things are going well with the relationship, but what happens when the new center of our universe does the unthinkable and breaks up with us? The odds are good that we'll lose our focus, and that the bottom will fall out of our perfect new world. Suddenly we're watching *Fatal Attraction* and craving rabbit stew. We go back to our old ways, analyzing every conversation we had with our new ex, thinking, "If only I'd done this or done that." Our insecurities come back with a vengeance, and the idea of taking a drink or a drug isn't usually far behind.

I know it's hard to stay out of the dating game, but try to remember that we're putting ourselves in a dangerous position when we get into new relationships that can leave us hurt. We don't know how to handle arguments and break-ups without alcohol or drugs, and we're going to be tempted to turn to using when things get rough. As with most of what's in this book, I had to learn things the hard way. Against the advice of many, I got into a relationship during early recovery, and when things went south, I went straight to the liquor store. I was one of these people who *always* drank when something went wrong with relationships, whether I broke it off or they did, but this knowledge didn't stop me from doing it. Mostly, it was because I craved the attention, no matter what the consequences.

I know from my own experience that it doesn't matter what people tell us concerning new relationships in early recovery. For the most part, we're just going to do what we are going to do. Still, if you have time for just one moment of clarity before going in for that kiss—or worse, leaping into the sack—use it to figure out which is your biggest priority, romance or recovery. More often than not we can have both, but early on, especially in the first year, it's not as easy as it sounds.

#7. Trigger Happy

In recovery, a *trigger* is usually a person, place, or thing that will set off an impulse or compulsion to use again. I had heard about triggers during one of my stints in rehab, along with the need to identify and avoid them at all costs. My biggest problem, it seemed, was that *everything* was a trigger to me. My spouse, my job, my family, the weather, days of the week ending with "y"...well, you get the idea. They were all triggers because they were just an excuse for me to drink.

When I finally got serious about getting sober, I was determined to make sobriety my number one priority. That meant finding my real triggers—not just the ones I wanted to hide behind—and then making some tough decisions. One of the hardest had to do with my sister. It happened, coincidentally, that we both got into recovery at around the same time. Despite the fact that she still lives in England, my country of birth, we had a long history of frequent phone calls. More often than not, we would both be drunk, idling away the hours together like two barflies sitting in the same booth, not two siblings seven time-zones apart.

With our sobriety on the line, however, the phone calls had to stop. There were simply too many familiar memories and sensations, too many patterns of behavior, to risk falling back into. With the trigger recognized, we both decided that it was for the best. It wasn't easy staying away from my closest friend and relative, but it was necessary for us two while we sorted our lives out. Later, when our heads had cleared a bit, we were able to pick things up where we left off. Now I talk to my sister all the time and we've visited each other more in the past two years than in the past twenty. Best of all, our conversations might still be crazy, and the text messages may sometimes say "My hamsters are back," but at least they aren't just drunken ramblings. Without a bottle between us, we've become closer than ever.

If you know that talking to certain people on the phone, or seeing them in person, might set you off on an emotional rollercoaster, then stay away for a while. Waiting until you have enough time in recovery to know how to cope with the people who push your buttons (family members can be especially strong triggers) isn't going to be easy, but it just might save the relationship, not to mention your life.

Staying away from people you used to drink or use with, along with the places where you did it, is also a good strategy. For me, this actually wasn't that difficult. I had long since stopped drinking socially in bars and clubs, so I tended to drink alone at home. Sure, I didn't have any friends left, but at least I didn't have any locations to avoid either. So, you see, there's a silver lining in everything.

In my earlier attempts at sobriety, when I still had friends and other hindrances to my drinking, I did find it hard to stay away. I'd been a keen pool player and was on a league at a local bar. I loved going out for a few games, so I tried going a couple of times without drinking, but it just wasn't the same. It wasn't long before I wanted to join in the fun, to have a drink and be one of the gang. In the end, I learned that I couldn't have both. I needed to either find a new scene, or stumble in my recovery.

If your friends are truly friends and not just fellow "barflies," they'll respect what you are trying to do. Suggest meeting for coffee, a movie, or dinner instead of a night on the town visiting bars and clubs. The first few times, they'll probably try to get you to come along to your old hangouts. Don't let temptation get the best of you. Recovery is all about now—what you do in this moment. You can't dwell on the past, remembering the times you were out living it up with your friends. You can acknowledge that there may have been good times, but in doing so you also need to acknowledge all the bad times too. Most alcoholics and addicts have plenty of those—enough to know they need to stay away from their triggers.

Remember that the craving and obsession are both very strong in the beginning of recovery and that *anything* can be a trigger if we let it. Protect yourself from people, places, and things that can set you off by staying away from them, at least for the first few months.

#8. Relapse

Someone once told me that I'd never have to drink or drug again, once I'd decided to quit. It didn't take me long to come up with a mental response: "Wow, really? Why don't you take that golden nugget of wisdom and shove it up your ass. That's really easy to say, but if it's true and we never have to drink or drug again, then why do so many people relapse?"

The truth, as I knew even then, is that it isn't as easy as that. We never completely beat our addiction; we just stay on top of it, day by day. To draw a clearer analogy, I think of my disease like a sleeping tiger: patient, cunning, and deadly. Even though we're no longer putting our drug of choice in our bodies, it lays quiet and still, waiting until we become exposed. Its patience is unrivaled, because it doesn't care how long it takes; it can wait days, months, even years. But sooner or later, it will see a weakness that makes us vulnerable. That vulnerability can manifest itself in a number of ways, but it usually includes being hungry, angry, lonely, tired, restless, irritable, or discontented (see Chapter 21, "H.A.L.T." for more on this).

Our disease knows when we are feeling any of these emotions and starts to plant ideas in our heads (the mental part of our problem). It tells us that we deserve to go out and have some fun, or that our drinking wasn't as bad as we thought it was. Surely, it says, we can have one drink and then stop. The disease knows our Achilles' heel, and it preys on the knowledge that controlling our drinking is the obsession of every alcoholic. Before we know it, the tiger is stirring. It's awake and pacing obsessively, in our minds, round and round in a circle. The hunt is on because the obsession has begun. The disease has its prey within reach. All it needs to do is wait, and our minds will take care of the rest.

This is what many call "the jumping-off point." It's where we either jump and relapse, or choose to fight. For me, the way to fight was with a program of recovery. I had jumped every time things had become difficult in the past. I had no protection from the disease; I was left wide open. Trying to stop drinking or drugging using willpower alone might work for a while, but our enemy knows our weaknesses and this defense will not last. One of my good friends in recovery, Mark S., says it best: *"Remember that our disease is our enemy and it wants us dead—but it will settle for having us drunk or high."*

A recovery program gives us tools to use, which we need to use before we get to the point where the tiger is stirring and the disease is awake. Having a system in place allows us to recognize negative feelings and protect ourselves by becoming mentally and spiritually fit. That way, when we inevitably let our guard down, there are backups in place. There are friends we can call, recovery meetings we can go to, or even books we can read.

The best defense is a good offense, and that's what a recovery program is. While it's true that relapse may be a very real *possibility*, it doesn't have to become a *reality*. Since working on my sobriety in a structured program, I have gone from having a relapse every couple of months to spending over two continuous years in recovery. And for this drunk, that's nothing short of a miracle.

#9. Fuck Your Feelings

Once, in a recovery meeting, I mentioned I was feeling miserable. I wasn't really expecting a response, but I got one anyway. From the other side of the room came the words that inspired this chapter: "Fuck your feelings."

As you might have guessed, my first instinct was to walk over to my vocal new friend and show my appreciation with a swift punch to the face. Instead, though, I just listened as he went on to explain what he meant by it. To my surprise, the whole thing began to make more sense.

Basically, in the first few months of recovery we don't know our heads from our asses. We tend to think we're fine, since we're no longer using, but our moods show us where our minds really are. We tend to yo-yo between extremes, like characters from a Winnie the Pooh book. One minute we're gloomy like Eeyore, and the next minute we're like Tigger, full of energy and bouncing off the walls.

We definitely tend to wear our feelings on our sleeves, finding it impossible to hide when we are mad, sad, or glad. But a feeling, *any feeling*, is an emotion, nothing more and nothing less. Emotions live in our heads, not in the real world. Today might *feel* like a Friday to me, but if my calendar says Tuesday, then that's the reality. What it feels like to me is irrelevant. The fact that I feel something doesn't make it real.

It's no different with our moods. If we're feeling sad or overcome with negative thoughts, we have to recognize them for what they are: *feelings*. They come and go for all people, whether they're in recovery or not. Normal people deal with them every day, without mind-altering substances. As addicts, we aren't normal and our tendency is to let these feelings run wild in our minds until we break down and use.

After my initial resentment toward this person who I believed had dismissed my feelings as meaningless, I realized he had just been trying to tell me that I didn't need to react immediately to my feelings and that I could in fact ride them out. When I started to feel sad, angry, or melancholy, I could simply say, "Fuck off! This is just a feeling. It will pass, I don't have to drink or use because of it." It didn't mean that my feelings weren't important; it just meant that I couldn't afford to get caught up in the extreme ups and downs that inevitably happen to all of us early on.

For those critical first few months of recovery, I decided to adopt this approach. I knew there would come a time when I could address these feelings that kept surfacing and put them to rest for good. That time did come (see Chapter 46, "Resentment"), and thankfully I had enough recovery under my belt by then to cross that bridge when I came to it.

#10. Reactions
From Others

for alcoholics and addicts in early recovery, it's an enormous accomplishment to have gone through another day clean and sober, mainly because we know firsthand how hard it is. We remember too clearly how it used to be: We'd start a new day with a sincere promise that things were going to be different, telling ourselves and anyone who would listen that we wouldn't use today, only to find two or three hours later that we were smashed, or high as a kite. This isn't a matter of being weak; this is part of our disease— the part that fucks with our minds and tells us we can drink or use successfully "just this one time." This is the insanity of our illness that normal people are unable to understand and identify with. It's a good idea to keep that in mind as you deal with the people in your life.

Sometimes normal people have a very hard time with the concept of addiction being a disease. They simply can't understand our state of mind and our actions because they are not alcoholics or addicts. They are not wired like we are. It's impossible for them to comprehend why we would risk losing everything over and over again, so they end up seeing us as selfish, compulsive, and irresponsible.

When you look at it from their point of view, it's easy to see why they are unable to share our enthusiasm for another day clean and sober. They do it every day, without giving it a second thought, and without a pat on the back. Going twenty-four hours without ruining their lives isn't a big deal, so we can't expect them to throw a parade each time we do it, nor can we make them understand how difficult it is for us those first few months. All we can do is go about our recovery with humility and recognize our own accomplishments within ourselves and with our peers. After a while, our "normal" family and friends might come to learn a little more about our disease, but in the meantime, we can't let it get to us. Our recovery is our business, and what other people think of us is not.

Some of the people who knew us while we were using will not know how to respond to our sobriety. Sometimes, these are our drinking or drug buddies who are still using themselves. No matter how close the bond seemed when we were under the influence, this might have been all we had in common with them. Now, with a clear head, we can recognize their sickness— the same one we're trying to beat—and the need to distance ourselves from them.

At the same time, you might have family members who won't understand your recovery, or what it means. They think now that you have stopped using alcohol or drugs, you're "all better." They imagine your problem is fixed, and that everything can now go back to normal, whatever that was. Or, even worse, they might feel like you're never going to be fixed, and that things can't ever go back to normal. Since they don't understand the mind of an addict and probably never will, all we can do is tell them what we have learned about our disease and that we need to work at it daily to stay healthy. Over time, by developing a routine and staying clean and sober, you might just win back their trust.

No matter how your loved ones react to your recovery, it's important to realize that they might need help too. It's not unusual for the people in an addict's life to have become co-dependent. A co-dependent is usually someone very close to us, like a spouse, a parent, or a best friend, who has been there to pick up the pieces for us when we've screwed up. They may have gotten so used to living each day on eggshells, changing their plans depending on what theatrics we pulled for the day, that they feel displaced and unsure of how to handle our newfound calm and independence. Luckily, there are places they can turn for help. Programs like Al-Anon (see "Recovery Resources" in the back of the book) hold meetings that can allow them to talk with others who have been through that before. We are not easy people to live with, especially during our using days and in early recovery, and it's important that our loved ones get a chance to look after themselves. That's what these programs offer.

As alcoholics and addicts, we have a support system in our recovery. Our friends and meetings help us to stay on stable ground, and it's important to encourage our family and friends to have the same foundation. You aren't going to get well alone, and they shouldn't have to either.

#11. Substituting and Fixing

it's common for addicts and alcoholics early in recovery to fixate on a person or activity as a substitute for drugs or alcohol. In other words, we try to plug the giant-sized hole inside us that we used to fill with our drug of choice. Often, what we try to fill it with is just as destructive as the substances we just cut out. As we adjust to our new sober lives, it's only natural that we find new ways to have fun and let off steam. The trouble comes when we revert back to our old tendencies, trading one compulsion for another.

For instance, it's not uncommon for both women and men in recovery to go on spur-of-the-moment shopping sprees, spending money on things they either don't need or can't afford. There's a certain rush we get from blowing a bunch of cash on jewelry, clothes, electronics, or even a new car, and it seems like a great way to reward ourselves for "good behavior." But what might seem like normal behavior is really just seeking instant gratification the same way we did when we used alcohol or drugs. The only difference is that instead of hitting the bottle, downing a few pills, or picking up a pipe, we're "using" through a new pair of shoes or a flat screen television.

Just like our "real" addiction, this type of habit will never leave us feeling satisfied. A friend of mine was prone to shopping sprees and compulsive spending. He had all the gadgets, electronics, cars, and other toys that a person could ever want or need. The fact that he couldn't really afford such a lifestyle was a minor detail. One day, we were talking about recovery over lunch. He told me that even though he appeared content on the outside, he never really felt satisfied and truly believed he could never be happy. I didn't see him for a long time after that, and when I ran into him again he told me he had relapsed and was using. The point is that shopping, or having lots of new things, will never work as a substitute for curing your real problems. If anything, such behaviors are likely to aggravate your troubles by putting you in debt.

As I mentioned earlier in the book, another way that we tend to get a fix is through relationships. There's an adrenaline rush that comes from the thrill of the chase, and a high you get from being in love. Once we win over our new conquests, though, we're hooked again, and suddenly our happiness depends on theirs. We begin looking to the other person's mood as a gauge for our own. We are only content if they are, and we'll do anything to keep the "love buzz" going. Sooner or later, though, the excitement dissipates, and when it does, we come back down to earth with a bump. We realize that this particular person can't make us happy, but because we aren't aware that people can't fix us, we start looking for the next person and the cycle begins again.

Food is another popular substitute, especially if we're prone to "emotional eating"—grabbing the nearest candy bar or tub of ice cream after a particularly grueling day. Like the other substitutes, binge eating might give us a sugar rush and a brief sense of satisfaction, but we'll soon come down from it feeling more lethargic and down in the dumps than we did before we ate.

While it's perfectly fine to treat ourselves to something nice once in a while, we are headed for trouble when we regularly use an activity or a person as a way to fix our mood. The excitement is fleeting, but the emotional and material cost certainly isn't, and no amount of shopping, sex, or food can fill the void that alcohol or drugs once filled. Whether we like it or not, the journey of recovery is about *self*-discovery. When we look outside of ourselves to other people and material things for happiness and fulfillment, we're looking in the wrong direction and asking for trouble.

#12. Isolating

if I had a dollar for every alcoholic and addict who ever said they spent too much time alone, I'd probably be able to afford that new liver by now. Isolating ourselves is what we do. We are the hermit crabs of our society, tucked inside the safety of our shells and oblivious to life outside of them.

Over the years, I've heard many people share stories from the end of their drinking and drugging careers. Most of them preferred to drink or use alone. Even if they'd once been social, spending their time at bars and parties, their habits became more and more focused on getting drunk or high as quickly as possible. With the pretense of socializing removed, they no longer wanted other people around to interfere with the process. At the same time, no one wanted to be around them while they were using anyway, so they were bound to end up alone, whether they wanted to or not.

In fact, if our isolation wasn't so pathetic, it would almost be funny. Not long ago, I was talking with some of my friends in recovery about how we'd used our walk-in closets (wardrobes in the UK) as a place to go and drink alone. That's about as isolated as you can get, spending time in a small, dark space just to hide what you're doing. Amongst our group, bathrooms, basements, attics, and even the crawl space under the house (I'm not that tall) were also fan favorites.

Sure, it sounds crazy now, but the fact is that we'd do anything to get away from the world. Unfortunately, it's a habit that we tend to carry over into our sober lives. And why shouldn't we? More often than not, we've alienated our family and friends, letting them down time and again. Besides, most of us have no idea how to act without our drugs of choice, having used them for so long to cover up our fears and anxieties about what other people might think or say.

It's no surprise, then, that we don't become social animals right away. Early on, most of us would super-glue our crab shells shut if we could. If we go to recovery meetings, we tend to walk in with our heads down, sit in the back, and do our best to become invisible. I know, because I've done it, just like 99% of the other alcoholics and addicts. I've yet to see a newcomer barge into a meeting, brimming with confidence and coolness (unless they're still drunk or high, which does happen now and again).

So how do you introduce yourself back into the land of the living? First off, be careful in terms of the activities you choose. You may still have friends who go out to bars and clubs, but you should think carefully before going to those places, for obvious reasons. There might come a time when you feel okay hanging out with other people who are drinking, but for the first year it's a good idea to pass. Also, being a designated driver for your friends can sound harmless, but bear in mind that you'll still have to go into the bars with a bunch of drunken people and then ferry them around town all night. Personally, I'd rather bash myself in the head with a brick, but that's just me. Going for a meal with friends tends to work out better, and if the others want to continue the party afterward, you can always go home once the meal is over.

Another way to get out there without endangering your sobriety is to expand your social circle. Obviously, if you go to recovery meetings, you'll meet all kinds of people. I'll be spending a lot of time talking about this in a bit, but for now let me just point out that recovery groups are always having social get-togethers, like BBQ's, game nights, potlucks, and so on. You might feel a little awkward going to them at first, but the good news is that you won't be alone—you'll be surrounded by other people who are feeling just as self-conscious as you are!

One other social event you'll invariably hear about is the sober dance. If you are one of these people who were comfortable dancing without alcohol or drugs, you might really enjoy these events. Everyone is different; personally, I'd rather have a root canal. I used to attend them, because I felt like I should go along with my new friends in recovery, but the whole thing felt like some torturous rite of passage from my teenage years. It was uncomfortable, irritating, and not my idea of a good time, so eventually, I just started skipping them to have coffee or dinner with friends who felt the same way I did. But, by all means try them for yourself before you dismiss the idea altogether. Live and let live!

The point here is that you should make an effort to be social for the sake of both your recovery and your mental health, but it's important that you find new ways that work for you. You don't have to prove anything by doing things you don't enjoy. Stick with the people who like the things you do. If you'd rather be at a movie than doing the electric slide, that's perfectly fine. After all, sobriety is about getting comfortable with who we are, and making decisions based on what's best for our recovery.

#13. "Firsts" in the First Year

as you start to build some time in recovery, there will be many "firsts." For instance, there's the first holiday season. Whether you celebrate Christmas, Kwanza, or Hanukkah, this can be a dangerous and precarious time. Alcoholics and addicts of every faith have long seen any holiday on the calendar as a reason to get drunk or high, from Groundhog Day to Saturday!

Not only are there the "recognized" public holidays to contend with, there are also personal milestones, such as birthdays and anniversaries, or family gatherings like weddings and funerals. There may also be relationship "firsts:" the first date, the first time we have sober sex, and even the first breakup. Everything feels new, and a little overwhelming. At least, I know everything felt this way to me. Up until I finally got sober, I had drunk my way through all of life's experiences, especially those red letter days when it seemed like the whole world was out having a party. So how did I get through them without drinking?

First, I faced up to the facts. I had been using holidays, like a lot of other things, as an excuse to drink. The idea that they were special days was a bit silly, since I was wasting them like I would any other. By choosing to stay sober, I was actually likely to have a better time celebrating a special day—or any day—than I had for a long while. And at the same time, I was making it easier on the people around me.

That brings us to a big part of the problem. Once we go into recovery, we tend to think we'll be the only ones not drinking at the big dinner or the cookout. Often, the fear of having to face people, and even worse, explain why we're not drinking or using, is enough to make us anxious and nervous before we even go anywhere. What do we talk about? How do we act? I remember going to my first holiday barbeque as a sober person feeling as though I were standing naked in a room of fully clothed people. I felt utterly exposed, completely convinced that everyone was talking about me and how bad it must be that I couldn't drink. If you find yourself with the same kinds of thoughts, let me fill you in. *Newsflash! Only alcoholics obsess about drinking.* Even when we aren't, we still think about other people's drinking— who's drinking what, and how much! Normal people don't give it a second thought, because they aren't alcoholics. *They don't care.* In fact, now that we are clean and sober, we might actually notice other people at parties, and how most of them sip their drinks slowly. As unbelievable as it sounds, we aren't really missing out on this orgy of booze and drugs. Most normal people actually only have one or two drinks, and then stop.

All that being said, there's no way around it—the first clean holiday party or sober family get-together can feel like walking the plank. So, first things first, have an escape plan, a way to leave the party if things become too overwhelming. Either bring your own car, or arrange for a ride home. Try to set yourself a goal: for example, that you'll stay until after the meal, or until a certain time when you know people will start letting loose. It's also a good idea to have phone numbers of sober people you can call in case you feel overwhelmed or uncomfortable. Having that encouraging voice on the other line can be a lifesaver when things get to be too much.

In fact, one of the best ways to combat the feeling of alienation we often experience at family or social events is to take along a sober friend. Having someone in the "trenches" with you is one of the most responsible actions you can do to safeguard your recovery and your state of mind. Having this person there can be a great psychological buffer, too. If the person you take with you does not know your family, he or she can keep an objective view of the situation and is less likely to put up with Uncle Bob's belligerent recollections of your most embarrassing moments. They can act like a shock absorber between you and a potentially uncomfortable situation.

Your first sober holidays are going to be stressful, but remember that you can get through them. Recognize a birthday or anniversary for what it is: a chance to reflect on the previous year and acknowledge how far you've come. In time, you will actually start enjoying those milestones instead of suffering through them.

#14. Dating in Early Recovery

i suspect that if we could go back in history and examine hieroglyphics from an ancient recovery meeting (if there were such a thing,) some version of *"Thou shalt wait to date"* would be on at least one of them. This has long been very sound advice for people who are early in sobriety, and for good reason.

Still, telling a person in early recovery to avoid dating for the first year is like telling a teenage girl she's too young to be interested in boys—you're betting against nature. We think that just because we aren't using anymore, we're ready to enter into all kinds of unions, from raunchy rendezvous to domestic bliss. We want to feel loved again, spiritually and physically, to have that wild fling or comforting caress. I know how strong the pull can be, but I also know how badly things can turn out.

That's because alcohol and drugs are just the tip of the iceberg for a lot of people. We may have stopped abusing our substance of choice, but our other problems are still there. On the one hand, we have our own emotional co-dependence to deal with. As I mentioned earlier in the chapter on substitution, we have a strong tendency to replace the highs and lows of using with the ups and downs of new relationships. That's nearly always a prescription for a relapse.

Even bigger than the threat to our sobriety is the one to our personal safety. Very often, men and women in recovery don't just decide to date; *They decide to date each other.* However, the mere fact that someone is in recovery doesn't make that person a saint. There are liars, sexual predators, abusers, thieves, and con-artists in our meetings, just as there are in the real world. They, like us, entered into their addictions with underlying problems.

During one of my failed attempts at sobriety, I met someone who hadn't had a drink in almost three years. I only had three months of sobriety myself, and anyone who could go a few years between cocktails was a winner in my book. It never entered my head that he could have other issues. We started a relationship, and although I had a weird feeling about him, I pushed it aside because I was getting attention. It felt great just to be wanted. However, his affection quickly turned to an unhealthy need for control, which erupted into heated arguments and subsequently led to both of us drinking. The first time he relapsed, he became violent in a way that I'd never imagined he was capable of. I was beaten black and blue, nursing a deep cut in my throat from being held down at knifepoint. It was a few days later, after being beaten unconscious numerous times, that I was finally able to escape to a safe house.

Looking back, I realize now that I was in no position psychologically to date. My judgment was clouded. I wasn't emotionally sober. "Emotional Sobriety" is a term that was coined by Bill Wilson, the co-founder of Alcoholics Anonymous, and in very basic terms it refers to our ability to recognize if we have an unhealthy dependency on another person or thing and therefore unhealthy expectations.

The problem was, I had no idea about any of this at the time and had already deemed myself ready to date. He could have been an ax murderer for all I knew, and it turned out that he very nearly was. But all I saw was a man with three years in recovery, and that amounted to an FBI background check in my mind. The weird feeling I had about him was an intuitive thought that was screaming, "This isn't right!" I chose to ignore it, though, so I could get my needs met.

You'd think I would have learned my lesson there, but I'm sad to say I didn't. After that train wreck of a relationship, I met another Mr. Wrong three months later. He was a man with more than four years of sobriety who seemed to be the poster child for a successful recovery program. The best part was that this superstar of sobriety *liked me*. We started dating, and after a few of months of sitting on a pink cloud, the shoe dropped. I found out that he'd been paying prostitutes for sex while he was seeing me, and for years before that. I ended the relationship, but not before I used his hooker fetish as an excuse to relapse.

I did, however, learn valuable lessons from those bad dating choices. People can give the illusion that they work a perfect program, but their actions will speak volumes about who they really are. It's a huge red flag if someone is still lying, cheating, and breaking the law while in recovery, because the very essence of every recovery program is honesty and integrity. Some people have some moral and behavioral issues that can't be fixed by simply putting down the alcohol or drugs.

It's true that we are sick people getting well, but some are sicker than others. When we're not yet well ourselves, we're hardly ready to judge who is safe and healthy and who isn't. I may have kissed my fair share of toads, but I wasn't any princess, either. Like attracts like—two sick people getting together does not make one healthy relationship. Keep this in mind as you consider dating in early recovery.

#15. Sober Sex

from the first time most alcoholics and addicts started having sex, booze or drugs were part of the package. Many of us should have been too young to be doing either, but we did both anyway. Over time, we started to associate one with the other, so that our addictive substance became not an addition to our sex life but a normal part of it. For me, drinking made me feel alive and uninhibited. It was the only way I could perform, because to me, that's what sex was—a performance, not an act of intimacy.

In speaking with other alcoholics and addicts, I found I wasn't alone. No matter where you are in recovery, sober sex is a big fear. With nothing to take away our inhibitions, we're left with little to shield us from our fears and insecurities. Sex is an interaction at the most personal level, something most of us have gone out of our way to avoid. Besides, there are so many things that can go wrong. For one thing, we're usually naked, which can be stressful in itself. What if our partner doesn't like the way we look? What if they don't think we're any good? It was easy to shut out these thoughts when we were using, but now they come flooding forward. When you think about it, sex is a bit like dancing—it's amazing that *anyone* can get through it without a few drinks. So how do we break our bad habits and get on with the business of getting it on?

Take a look back at your life and see if there's a pattern with regard to your drinking or drugging and what you've done between the sheets. I was very young when I became sexually active, and right from the start, I associated sex with being drunk or high. I felt like I needed booze to be intimate. If you've always relied on a substance to make your own sex life "go," now is a good time to confront that dependency head-on. Realize that it truly will be like the first time again in a lot of ways (awkward and over very quickly), but that things will get better from there.

It's been said that people who start using alcohol or drugs in their teens stop growing emotionally at that point, which means that although they experienced adolescence physically, they did not experience it emotionally. This rang true to me, at least when it came to getting physical, because now that I was sober I often felt like an embarrassed, fumbling teenager all over again. It's not unusual for people in recovery to act out emotionally as well, often mistaking lust for love, and we get hurt easily because we're still very naïve in a lot of ways.

The fact that we're older doesn't mean we're wiser, and rushing into any kind of relationship is risky, as I mentioned in the previous chapter. If you do decide to date in early recovery, though, don't sell yourself short by thinking you aren't worth waiting for. There are a lot of people, in and out of recovery, who might try to take advantage of you. How do you tell them apart? By doing things the old-fashioned way and spending time with them. You'll soon find out where their interests lie, because most people don't stick around for stimulating conversation if it's really just sex they want. We all deserve respect, and choosing to wait a while before jumping into bed with someone builds that, for both of you. Besides, the decision to wait will not only develop your self-esteem, it will also give you time to figure out if you actually *like* the other person first, a step most of us have skipped a time or two.

If you are already in a relationship when you get clean, and feel anxious or uncomfortable about having sober sex, talk to your partner about it. It's very important that you communicate what's going on, especially since you and your partner might be out of sync. Early recovery is extremely tough, and sometimes we don't feel very amorous in the first few months or so. Our moods can climb and fall so often that sex becomes the last thing on our minds. In fact, the emotional elements can even become physical. It's not uncommon for men and women in recovery to have problems climaxing because they feel self-conscious, or they're having trouble letting go. This awkwardness can be tough to work through, and most "experts" aren't a lot of help. I can remember looking through a few books on the subject, searching for a few tips to help me loosen up. The most common suggestion I found? Have a couple glasses of wine.

Obviously, drinking or drugs weren't an option for me, and they shouldn't be for you either. Put them out of your mind and do something else. There are a lot of ways to feel sexy together, and sometimes even simple things, like getting dressed up to go to dinner, can go a long way towards setting the mood. You could also do things the old-fashioned way, like you might have done in the beginning of your relationship. Holding hands, making out, or just staying up to talk can help you feel more intimate.

Since this isn't a book on foreplay, I'll stop there. But as you contemplate sober sex, remember the cardinal rule: It's all about being relaxed. The more confident in our sobriety and comfortable in our own skin we can become, the better things will go. Try not to stress out about it, because it's going to take some time. If you keep practicing and communicating your needs to your partner, though, you might stop worrying about sex and just enjoy it.

#16. Getting Honest

honesty really is the best policy.
However, although it may come naturally to
normal people, it can take some practice for the majority of
alcoholics and addicts. Most of us have spent a good deal of
our time trying to cover up our addiction, creating quite the web
of lies along the way. Dishonesty can be so ingrained in us that
sometimes we aren't even conscious that we're lying.

During my drinking days, I missed work a lot. Usually, I'd
call my boss with my latest fairy tale, complete with a plot,
a villain, and a damsel in distress (usually me). I just seemed
to have a natural ability to spout bullshit, and the worst part
was that I actually believed some of it myself. I told one of
the more deplorable of these lies about ten years ago. I was
broke, homesick, and missing my family in England, so my
mother agreed to buy me a ticket so I could come home for a
visit. Naturally, I booked the flight without giving it a second
thought. Later, after I'd already completed my arrangements, I
remembered that I'd have to say something to my employer. I
didn't think "I'm not going to come to work for ten days" was

going to cut it, so I marched in the next day and told my boss that my dad had been run over by a car. Obviously, I'd need to go home and tend to things.

I remember feeling guilty at the time, but not enough to stop me from going. In my mind, the lie was necessary and justified. That was how I operated, doing or saying whatever I needed to in order to satisfy my selfishness. But this lie, like all the others I told, came with a hefty price. The guilt stuck with me for years, festering in the back of my mind, until I was finally able to address it and admit what I had done when I became sober (see Chapter 48, "Amends").

If we are honest with ourselves (yes, let's start now), dishonesty has most likely been part of our lives for as long as we can remember. It's wrapped up in the mental part of our disease. Long before I ever picked up my first drink, I lied to my school friends about my dysfunctional family members and their substance abuse. Then, in adolescence, I lied about my own substance abuse to my teachers and friends. In adulthood, I continued telling lies to my family, friends, and employers to cover up my out-of-control behavior and avoid the consequences.

Dishonesty is part of our past, whether we like it or not. While we can't change what we did, we can certainly do things differently from now on. The first step is to start being completely honest in all areas of our lives. For one thing, telling the truth is the right thing to do, and that really should be reason enough. If it isn't, though, remember that dishonesty is a threat to your recovery. As alcoholics and addicts, we can't afford to harbor the guilt that comes from lying, because it will eat away at our conscience and take us right back to our drug of choice.

A good way to start is by checking your motives when making decisions. For instance, if you're planning on doing something, ask yourself this question before you act: *What am I hoping to get out of this?* This can help you to be honest in all areas of life. Suppose you want to ask someone out for coffee, offer someone a ride, or volunteer to babysit for a friend. These are all normal, everyday situations, and you might not think you have any agenda at all. But often, deep within our diseased minds, an ulterior motive can be found. For instance, the person you ask out for coffee is a friend of someone you are interested in romantically and you want to find out more about them. Or, maybe you've offered that ride so you can ask a favor in return, and the real reason you offered to babysit was because your friend has access to the Internet at home and you don't.

Of course, you might not have any dark reasons for the things you do. Most of us, even the worst substance abusers, aren't criminal geniuses or malicious masterminds. The point isn't that you're always going to do or think something wrong; it's that you need to prevent yourself from slipping up before you start. Remember, if we're dishonest, selfish, or manipulative from the start, chances are we won't feel good later, even if we do get the results we wanted.

Another way to be honest is by telling people we are in recovery. That's not to say we need to send out a mass e-mail or anything, but rather, that we need to acknowledge that it's nothing to be ashamed of. Besides, chances are that people have known about our substance abuse problem long before we came to do anything about it. Most of us have wreaked a path of destruction before we sobered up that hasn't gone unnoticed.

When I finally got serious about my sobriety, I didn't care who knew, and I decided I wasn't going to lie anymore. I even told the tax man! I was on the phone setting up a payment plan, and I mentioned that my lack of prior payments was largely due to my out-of-control substance abuse problem. I went on to say that I'd turned my life around, and having achieved six months sober, I was now in a position to start working on my debt. He actually congratulated me, set up a payment plan for my balance, and wished me luck!

Some situations are more sensitive, like when you're dealing with an employer. Unless you are on the verge of being fired because of your substance abuse, it's really none of your employer's business. You should tell them if and when you feel the need to tell them, when you can't perform your job anymore, or when you need time off for recovery purposes. In many cases, know that your employer may be legally required to allow you to get the treatment you need. And what's more, they might be more understanding than you thought they would once you've told them the truth about your condition. Whatever you decide, if you stay with your recovery program, your boss will likely notice sooner rather than later that your job performance and attendance have improved. People in recovery often turn out to be very reliable and efficient employees, once we finally get our acts together.

If you continue to practice honesty, you'll be amazed at how liberating it is. Before long, you'll stop feeling trapped by lies and deceit. You'll sleep well at night and wake up with a clean slate each morning. The best part is, once you realize how good it feels to be honest, keeping it up becomes natural.

#17. If It's Broken, Fix It!

We alcoholics and addicts tend to take everything way too personally. When we get hurt by someone, we have a hard time letting it go, even if we've gotten an apology from this person. If you haven't guessed by now, learning not to get hung up on things is an important part of the recovery process. We might not be able to forget at first, but we need to get good at the forgiving. But what happens when the shoe is on the other foot, when we're the ones causing the harm?

One of the best pieces of advice I ever got, concerning my recovery, was to "keep my side of the street clean." In other words, if I made a mess, I had to take care of it right away. There is no room in our lives for the feelings of guilt and remorse that come after a fight with a loved one or a run-in with a co-worker. Holding onto those feelings will only leave us with an unresolved issue. No matter how small each one might be, with enough time, it can lead to a relapse. Working in tandem, lots of them will almost certainly destroy our sobriety.

Normal people tend to address confrontation right away. Apologizing and getting over things comes naturally to them. We are not normal, though, and procrastination and avoidance are our natural tendencies. For most of my life, I avoided taking responsibility for any conflict or misunderstanding. I would walk away from a friendship or a relationship before I'd admit to my part in a problem, because there was no way I was going to look soft or weak. When I first practiced addressing my wrongs as soon as they occurred, it felt completely foreign to me. After the original awkwardness, though, this new way of living proved to be much different than what I thought it would be like. Instead of appearing weak when I admitted I was wrong, I actually felt good.

I remember working once in a small office with a woman I couldn't stand. She had a personality that grated on me like fingernails down a chalkboard. We were complete opposites. One day, we got into it over something trivial, and during the argument, I became overly rude and critical. Had this happened when I was drinking, I would have been pleased that I'd gotten the better of her and won the argument. As a result of my recovery program, though, I was really trying to do things differently. I guess it must have worked. That night I couldn't stop thinking about the quarrel, and even though I still couldn't stand this other woman, I felt awful. The next morning I went into the office and apologized to her for my behavior. I admitted I'd been out of line and told her she didn't deserve to be spoken to in that way. She seemed a little shocked that I would apologize, but she accepted it anyway. And even though we were never going to be friends, working together was more tolerable after that.

There have been other transformations too. I can no longer walk away from a store or supermarket if I've been given too much change, or if the cashier forgot to charge me for something; I have to go back and pay for it or give the extra money back. This is from someone who had no problem stealing a Christmas tree (the cashier forgot to charge me for it; I realized the mistake outside of the store, but I took it anyway). There have been entire books and movies made about the kind of person who could steal a Christmas tree, so I think that incident says a lot about who I was back then.

Through my recovery program, though, I've learned to forgive others their wrongs, and to correct mine right away. As a side effect, I feel a lot better than I did back then. Obviously, I'm not perfect, but I'm working on being a better person, and that's all any of us can do.

When we are in the wrong, we must admit it and do our best to make things right. Not only does this show integrity, it's also important for our recovery. If we don't keep our conscience clear, we'll keep obsessing about it until we feel bad enough to pick up a drink or a drug. We need to keep our side of the street clean if we're to have any hope of doing the same for our bodies.

#18. Spouses and Partners

People say you need to put recovery above all else in your life, because if you don't have recovery, you won't have a life. This is very true early on, but make sure you talk to your spouse or partner before you dive in and exclude them completely. It's a good idea to explain to them that the first ninety days of sobriety are extremely crucial, and that you're going to need to dedicate a lot of time to your recovery. There's no doubt that this can be very hard on everyone, but it will be well worth it in the long run.

Your family may be a little put-off at first. It's natural for your family members to think that because you've stopped using, you'll immediately want to spend time with them. It's often difficult to balance our own needs with the needs of our loved ones. For that reason, it's common to hear of troubles in marriages and relationships in which one partner is an addict or alcoholic in recovery and the other isn't.

If this is the case in your relationship, begin by trying to look at things from the perspective of your partner. Most of us have been pretty selfish and self-centered. We've probably neglected and hurt them for months, or even years. Now they see us in recovery, feeling and looking better than we have in a long time, and they want to be around us. They want to be involved in our lives now that they can actually stand us.

A friend's husband told me that once his wife started recovery, he felt like he didn't know who she was anymore. She was never home, and when she was, she was always on the phone and text messaging her new sober friends. It was as if she were now addicted to recovery and had replaced the obsession of drinking with the obsession of not drinking. Moreover, she always made an extra effort to look nice when she went out. It didn't take long for him to become convinced she was having an affair. His wife's side of the story was that she was just enjoying her new life, her new friends, and the sense of independence that she hadn't had when she'd been using. She said that her husband was being too critical because he was used to her being a wreck, clinging to him and begging for forgiveness for her latest screw-up.

This situation is far from unusual, and it can cause countless arguments. One spouse is hurt and angry that they aren't being included, and the other retaliates by saying that their normal spouse just doesn't understand. This creates a bad situation for everybody. While there may be nothing going on romantically with our recovery friends, telling our significant others that they don't "get us" anymore only alienates them further. It is important to acknowledge our partners' needs as we go through recovery, they may not know firsthand the personal torment and hell that we've gone through like our new friends do, but haven't they gone through hell too?

It doesn't have to be a constant battle; there is a way to compromise. My friend started to make her husband feel included. She kept him clued-up about the meetings she was attending, and if she was going for coffee afterward, she invited him along. She also made a dinner date with a recovery friend and her husband (who were also going through a similar experience) so they could all get to know each other. And when she was alone with her husband, she turned off her phone and told her friends she'd be out of contact for the evening.

Even if it's for just a few hours each week to begin with, give your partner your exclusive attention. You'll be surprised at how a little goes a long way toward rebuilding your relationship and regaining trust. You can also read books together on recovery and look into family support groups such as Al-Anon. Your spouse doesn't have to go to these meetings, but encouraging and making him or her aware of these groups will show that you're thinking of his or her well-being too. My friend's marriage isn't perfect, but I don't know of one that is! The most important thing is that they're working on it together and not leading completely separate lives.

There are also, of course, situations in which both people in the relationship should be in recovery but only one of them is. If this is the situation you find yourself in, just keep working your program and be sure to ask your spouse if he or she would like to attend a meeting with you once in a while. It's very important, though, to remember that we can't force someone to get clean and sober (think of how we were). However, if your spouse sees you doing it, he or she may feel like trying it too, though don't set your hopes sky-high. Your spouse might refuse to go, or might try it and decide it's not for him or her. You probably didn't get sober overnight, and your spouse won't either.

In the event that your partner continues his or her substance abuse and has no desire to get clean and sober, you may need to consider moving to an alcohol and drug-free environment where you won't have to face the temptation on a daily basis. It's unfortunate, but it does happen. Often, leaving the person you're with can be a gut-wrenchingly painful decision. However, it also might be the best one you can make, for your sobriety and safety—and for your spouse's, too.

#19. Children

Our addictions have done damage to our relationships with our children. It's inevitable, but not irreparable. Whether we think we hid our habit from them or not, chances are we didn't. Children are very perceptive and we need to give them credit for that, even when we think they're too young to notice. When we stop using, they know there's something different about us—they might be too young to understand what it is, or why our behavior has changed, but they know that it has. We need to show them, with our actions, that we can act responsibly and consistently. This won't be easy, even if they're too little to remember exactly what happened. If you have older children who can remember what you were like when you drank or used, it's going to be even harder to rebuild that trust. It's by no means impossible, but it's going to take a lot of time and effort.

We can never reclaim the time we've wasted drinking and drugging. It's natural to feel regret for this, especially when we've chosen to get drunk or high instead of spending time with our kids. Some addicts will argue that they did spend time with their children, that they were "functioning" drunks or addicts, keeping up with their responsibilities in the home. Usually, though, they're fooling themselves. They might have been present physically, but mentally they were obsessed with their addiction. Imagining that their children didn't notice is wishful thinking, at best.

For the first four years of my son's life I battled unsuccessfully to stay sober. I was diagnosed with postpartum depression a few months after he was born, but the antidepressants I was taking didn't have a chance to work because I was drinking so heavily. My "World's Greatest Mom" credentials only snowballed from there: I spent my first Mother's Day alone because of a binge, and I spent my son's first birthday in a treatment center. Not surprisingly, his father filed for divorce and was given full custody. I was awarded visitations, but they were contingent on my staying away from alcohol.

After the divorce, I could only manage a few months sober at a time. A pattern emerged in which I'd see him regularly for a few months, relapse, and then only be in his life sporadically until I could piece my life back together. It wasn't until he was four years old that I finally made it through my first continuous year of recovery.

At the time, he obviously didn't understand why he lived with his dad and only stayed with me on weekends. He was confused and acted out, misbehaving and defying me at every possible turn. I realize now that he was testing to see how far he could push me before I'd take off again. Until I got serious about my recovery, my son had been on an emotional rollercoaster set in motion by my behavior for all of his young life. He needed reassurance that I'd be around for him, not just physically, but emotionally. The only way that I could regain his trust and prove to him that I wasn't going anywhere was to *show* him.

That meant providing stability and consistency. When I said I was going to do something, I made sure that I did it. If I said I'd call him on the phone, I *always* called. And if I promised to pick him up at 6:00, I showed up at 5:59. It didn't matter if my ass was falling off—I kept my word. There are no shortcuts to rebuilding trust, but honesty, reliability, and stability do work. I know because I did it. It wasn't easy, but I'm grateful every day for my son, who now shares his time equally between his father and me.

As I mentioned earlier, rebuilding relationships with older children can be more difficult. This is especially true for teenagers because, let's be honest, teenagers like to rebel against their parents in the first place, whether they have good reason or not. A friend of mine has four years of recovery, with a husband and a teen at home. Her daughter was eleven when she got sober, so she remembers her mother being drunk and the lifestyle that went with it. Even now, these memories are a constant source of problems between the two of them. While she's able to be in her daughter's life consistently now, there's still noticeable friction. Only time will heal the damage completely.

There are some very good programs for teenagers living in these situations, like Al-Ateen (see listings in back of book), where they can go and talk about their experiences with their peers. This is very important because they need to hear and be heard by other teens who have been in their shoes, rather than parents or adults, who might as well be from a different planet as far as they are concerned.

As you look to repair your relationships with your children, remember that the door swings both ways. It's not unusual for us to have inherited our problems from our own parents. Being the daughter of an alcoholic, my siblings and I grew up with the disease in our household. We experienced the constant feeling of "walking on eggshells" in our home, never knowing what to expect or how to act to avoid a scene. Our home life was anything but normal, but we didn't know any different. My father was a practicing alcoholic until the day he died, while my mother stopped drinking seven years ago. At thirty-four years old, I was supposed to be a grown woman when my mother got sober, but my age didn't stop me from blaming her for my awful childhood. I still remembered all the bad times, and I made sure she'd never forget, either. But with time, and my own experiences in recovery, I learned to let go of some of that hurt. Now, my mother and I have a better relationship than we ever did, or probably could have had otherwise. It isn't only that we both no longer drink; it's that we no longer dwell on the past, so we're able to enjoy the present. I love and appreciate my mother for who she is today, not for the image I had of her as a kid.

It doesn't matter what age our children are when we get sober. Whether they're three, thirteen, or thirty, our recovery can be the cornerstone of a new relationship with them. Obviously, the younger your kids are, the less likely they'll remember your "using" days, but that doesn't mean you can't get close to them at any age. Sometimes, as with me and my mother, remembering the bad times help us to appreciate the good ones, and in doing so, we can all move on and begin to heal. It's true that the age of our children is a key factor in how they deal with our newfound sobriety, but if we make an effort to be accountable and present in their lives, the relationship will get a chance to rebuild itself and ultimately grow no matter how young or old they are.

#20. I Want It and I Want It Now!

Patience is a virtue that most alcoholics and addicts simply don't have, and once we start to feel better physically and emotionally, it only gets worse. We think that because we've quit using, we can take on the world and make things magically better in no time flat. But, as you'll undoubtedly hear a thousand times in recovery, "We didn't get sick overnight, so we shouldn't expect to get well overnight either." If you're like me, you'll hate hearing that! After my first few months, I was feeling better and working hard at my recovery. I wanted my new and improved life right away! But Rome wasn't built in a day (another one of those sayings), and our new lives won't be either.

One of the areas where we have to be patient is in rebuilding relationships. We know we've changed, but other people need time to adjust. With all the broken promises and lies most of us have doled out over the years, can we really blame people for not wanting to listen and take us seriously? Over time, the people we live and work with have grown immune to the things we say we're going to do. The only way to convince them we're serious is with action. I know that after years of selfish behavior, meaningless promises, and habitual relapses, no one had time for my latest attempts at sobriety. When I finally got serious about cleaning up, I knew I had to stop talking about it and just do it.

By the same token, we have to be patient with ourselves. Getting sober is a bit like skydiving or swimming with the sharks—it isn't quite as effortless as it looks in the brochures. It's easy to get despondent. Early on, there were days when I would cry over nothing, followed by days when I couldn't stop being angry with myself for the years I'd wasted. Highs and lows are a natural part of any life, especially in recovery, but this knowledge doesn't help when we keep asking ourselves, "Why don't I feel better? Does it have to take so long? Is this going to be worth it?"

As addicts and alcoholics, we always want the "quick fix"—it's our nature. It's the reason we used substances to feel anything other than what we were feeling. But there is no quick fix for what we are going through; we just have to do it. It all comes back to staying in the day we are in, and not worrying about the future or dwelling on the past. Instead of worrying about tomorrow, be responsible *today* and make the right choices. Get to work on time, spend time with your kids or spouse, or meet with another recovering addict. It's only by doing the day-to-day things we take for granted that we can get back into mainstream life.

When we stop expecting applause and recognition in return for our recovery, miracles will start to happen. I'm not talking about burning bushes, but rather the miracle of regaining peoples' trust. For me, it happened when my ex-husband agreed to let our son stay overnight with me for the first time in a very long while. I hardly had any furniture, and no TV, but it was a miracle to me and it symbolized a whole new beginning for us. Sure, this transition didn't happen overnight, and I had to earn my ex-husband's trust back bit by bit, but this was something he'd told me would never happen. And after doing things the right way, one day at a time, here it was happening! I remember feeling overwhelmed with gratitude for my sobriety, and for the opportunities that were presenting themselves to me because of it.

Life is about the small stuff we put together to make up the big picture. If we're patient, concentrate on the little things, and continue keeping our word, the rest will fall into place. These miracles can happen to all of us. All we have to do is suit up and show up on a daily basis.

#21. H.A.L.T.

remembering this acronym—
Hungry, Angry, Lonely, Tired—is easy enough, but using it in our everyday lives is a bit tougher. That's because it's common to feel any or all of these emotions in early recovery, and it's very important for alcoholics or addicts to keep our feelings in check. The tendency for most of us has always been to act *now* and think *later*, letting any awkward or unpleasant emotion become an excuse to drink or use. To overcome these bad habits, especially early on, we need to stop the problem at its source.

With that in mind, H.A.L.T. is regularly used in recovery programs as an effective way to make us stop and take time to identify the cause of a feeling, so we can deal with it right away. This is no small feat, considering that we've relied on drugs and alcohol to crush down feelings of anger and frustration. Left unattended, just one of them could lead to a relapse.

Even worse, it can happen out of the blue. There we are one minute, coasting through the day, when out of nowhere an incident throws us off our game. It may be something or nothing. Maybe a person makes an offensive comment at work, a phone call brings some bad news, or we just get cut off in traffic. Normally, we might get a little upset, but then we let it go without much thought. If we aren't feeling too well emotionally or physically, though, our addict minds can latch onto negative emotions and turn something insignificant into a crisis that we think only drink or drugs will ease.

This was the case for me not long ago when a guy who worked in a coffee shop was really rude to me. At the time, I felt as though I'd been treated unfairly and almost said something to him about it. Instead, I chose not to and left. Later that night, I couldn't stop thinking about the incident. I was so angry that someone would treat me that way that I kept running the whole incident through my head, over and over. My anger was fueled more from being very tired, though, than from the slight itself. The next morning, well rested, I had breakfast and coffee and felt like myself again. In fact, I didn't think once about the rude coffee shop guy (that is, until I drove by the shop, and then I felt like throwing a brick through the window!). In the end, though, I realized that I had just been very tired, and that fatigue had caused me to start thinking obsessively and to conjure up an impression that really wasn't as bad as I had thought.

Often, if we ask ourselves, "Am I Hungry, Angry, Lonely, or Tired?" we can identify the root of our feeling and give ourselves time to remedy the problem. The problem wasn't some guy who was rude, or some woman who cut you off three lights back—it's that you skipped breakfast or didn't sleep well last night, or that you're angry because you're running late. Once we realize that we are reacting to one of these feelings, we can stop, reboot ourselves, and get back on track. Be responsible for your well-being and take action. If you are cranky and tired, get a cup of coffee or grab a snack. Then, when you're at home later, look after yourself. Take a bath and have a good meal, or call a friend to vent your anger if things are still bugging you.

It's very important that we look after our bodies, minds, and spirits. We can help our bodies by sticking to a daily schedule, eating regularly, getting some exercise, and going to bed at a similar time each night. In the same way, working through a recovery program will help in healing your mind and spirit by helping you to regain balance and put things in perspective. Eventually, you'll feel less put out by life's smaller irritations. In the meantime, though, adopting H.A.L.T. as a gauge of your feelings might just alleviate a lot of your pain and drama before it has a chance to happen.

#22. Depression

It's common to feel down or even depressed in the early months of recovery; after all, we have taken away the alcohol and drugs, the one thing we counted on to lift or change our mood.

I'm not going to go into detail about the scientific reasons why recovering alcoholics and addicts are prone to depression, because when we first get clean and sober, most of us don't care about the serotonin and dopamine levels in our brains, or how and why they became depleted. How our neurotransmitters got damaged doesn't make a blind bit of difference if we feel like throwing ourselves off a bridge. All we know is that when we're going through it, we feel like shit.

On a more basic level, though, the problem is easy to understand. We have self-medicated for so long that we really don't know how to feel, making any minor emotion seem unbearable without our "little helper." I'm certainly not a medical professional, and I wouldn't be able to diagnose you through a book if I was, so I'm not about to tell you all about your mental state. That's a job for your own physician, and it's not a bad idea to have your doctor examine you. I have experienced it for myself, though, having been diagnosed with postpartum depression and medicated for four years. I stopped taking medication three years ago, though, so I've seen life in recovery from both sides of the fence—with medication, and without.

Some of you reading this may have been prescribed medication for depression while you were still using. If this is the case, then most likely the treatment didn't get a chance to work, as alcohol or drugs interfere with a medication's effectiveness. Once I stopped using alcohol, I found that the pills worked and I felt better. No longer drinking, I continued to take antidepressants for a few months and saw my doctor regularly. After some time had passed, I spoke to him about coming off the antidepressants and he agreed to lower the dose over a period of a few months. We kept this up until I eventually stopped taking them completely.

I've heard of some people in recovery (thankfully only very few) who believe that antidepressants are mood-altering drugs, and that therefore taking them while being in recovery equates to not being clean and sober. This is both ill-informed and dangerous. As with most things, it's likely that the ones making the fuss have never experienced depression themselves. It goes without saying that you should *never* discontinue your medication just because of some comment made by a friend or someone you listened to in a recovery meeting.*

Depression is a disease, just like addiction, and left untreated it will only get worse. A friend in recovery mentioned in a meeting that he was feeling a bit down. I talked to him afterward, and he said he couldn't shake this downer he was on but hadn't seen a doctor yet. I made a joke and told him that I'd better not hear about him drinking or I'd kick his ass. He said he wouldn't drink. I'm sorry to say that I never saw him again, because he committed suicide a week later. His autopsy showed he was clean and sober when he died, but this man obviously wasn't healthy mentally.

It's common in early recovery to feel sad or withdrawn, and this may last for a day or two before it passes. However, if the symptoms persist for a week or more, it's imperative that you seek advice from a medical professional. Depression is every bit as serious as addiction, but luckily, you don't have to fight either of them alone.

You should never stop taking anti-depressants without consulting your doctor first.

#23. The Medical Profession

Last year I was fortunate enough to hear a doctor speak to a room full of recovering alcoholics and addicts. What he said changed my attitude toward the medical profession, and particularly what I thought about their disdain for "our kind."

Before hearing this doctor talk, I had my own ideas of how they viewed us. My beliefs were fueled by my own experiences with my family doctor, along with professionals in various treatment centers, detox units, and hospital emergency rooms. I felt sure most medical personnel looked at us as lost causes, and the doctor I heard speak that day confirmed that they did indeed think that. However, they have good reason to think this way, which I realized when he went on to explain his statements further. Apparently, in the medical community, we alcoholics and addicts have a reputation for being extremely flakey (who'd have thought that?). Besides being hard to treat, success rates are notoriously low. We seldom give the medical professionals who see us any proof that we can and do recover, so why should we be surprised when they think it doesn't happen? After all, medicine is a science, and scientists require proof to demonstrate a theory. The problem is that we are the proof, and most of us have failed to tell the truth so often to our doctors that they don't know what to believe anymore.

I know I lied to different doctors and caregivers about how much booze I used to consume, and I've got plenty of friends in recovery who did the same. Our doctors have heard all about how we're "recreational users," how we only have a couple of drinks on the weekend, and how we have never tried any illegal drugs, and they have spotted time and time again our attempts to lie about our family histories.

Even when we are honest, admitting to our doctor that we may have a substance abuse problem usually amounts to nothing. We tend to listen to their advice for treatment and reply, "Thanks, but I think I'll try it my way first," promising to let them know how we get on. But, as usual, we fail to keep our word and don't see them again for months, if ever, so all they remember of us is that we were practicing alcoholics or addicts. No wonder the medical profession thinks we're lost causes! Even if we do go on to live clean, sober lives, we don't bother to go back and tell them how we did it; we just move on and forget the part when we showed up at the doctor's looking like a wreck and acting like a loon.

The doctor who I heard speak was the founder of the Alcohol and Addiction unit of a psychiatric hospital. He talked about it being our responsibility to educate the medical profession about how we got clean and sober and how we are able to stay that way. The tactic we need to use to educate them is simple: We need to deploy a *show and tell* approach.

Regardless of how many weeks or months sober you have, it's a good idea to go and see your doctor for a check-up, let them know you are in recovery, and tell them that you'll be back to see them with your progress in six months. Now here comes the hard part: *Keep your word and go and see your doctor in six months!* Rather than fading into the background, we should proudly go back to our doctors and say, "Look at me now!" (Keep in mind that you might look like a different person and may need to jog their memory!)

Too often, doctors see us fail. In order to keep some hope, they really need to see and hear some of the success stories, too. Once they see the evidence that recovery programs can work, they're able to do a better job for the next alcoholic or addict they see. By making this small visit, we are showing them living, breathing proof that recovery works. We can change the medical profession's perception of us and this disease, but it's up to us.

#24. Antabuse

You might have heard of people taking Antabuse (also called disulfiram) during early recovery. This is a medication sometimes prescribed by medical professionals to alcoholics to help them abstain from alcohol. It can also be court-ordered for the same reasons.

The drug works by interfering with the metabolism of alcohol in the liver, causing severe side effects to any drinking. Reactions can include painful headaches, vomiting, shortness of breath, red rashes over the face and neck, and heart palpitations.

Naturally, I took Antabuse a number of times at different stages in my alcoholism, although more often than not it usually wasn't my idea. The first time was to satisfy my family. The big problem with that was, I was not self-motivated, so I inevitably drank again. I'd read that I needed to wait two weeks after stopping the drug before drinking alcohol again, to be sure the medication was out of my system, but I knew there was no way I could wait that long. Five days after discontinuing the drug I played it "safe" and only took one shot of vodka. I figured I'd make sure I didn't notice anything too uncomfortable before

I started further into the bottle. Well, I definitely did notice *something*—that I thought I was going to die. The reaction was painful and terrifying. Within minutes of ingesting a solitary drink, my head was pounding unlike any headache I had ever had before. What's more, my face turned bright red, I was burning up, and my heart was racing. I felt as though I couldn't breathe, and I wanted to crawl out of my skin because it hurt so much. After a few moments I started vomiting and couldn't stop until it seemed like the alcohol was out of my system, but even then, I could barely move. The effects lasted until the next day, when I was finally able to get out of bed. I have no idea what would have happened if I had drank more than that one shot, but my excruciating experience didn't leave me all that curious, either. I vowed to never take it again.

My alcoholism caught up with me, and I was court-ordered back on the drug after I was arrested for drunk driving. This isn't normal for a first offense, but the court didn't see me as normal, possibly because at 110 pounds I'd drunk enough to render most people twice that size unconscious. The judge decided that if I was walking and talking with that much alcohol in my system, then I obviously had the kind of huge tolerance only seen in alcoholics. I was instructed to take the drug under supervision until I completed my alcohol education classes, which took nine months, and I remained sober during that time. When my probation had been satisfied, I came off the medication, but I was very nervous about it. For close to a year, it had been the only thing standing between me and a drink. With no other real recovery program in place, Antabuse was my program. It turned out my concerns weren't unfounded, because a couple of months later I drank again.

Everyone's experience is different, but for me, Antabuse was a short-term solution. If you are going to take it, you *have* to be self-motivated, because if you drink the consequences are very painful and sometimes even deadly. There are other risks, too. Anything containing alcohol—hairspray, perfumes, cough medicines, mouthwash, nasal sprays, cold remedies, and so on—can cause severe reactions. Choosing whether to try it or not is not a decision to be taken lightly, and you should talk it over with your doctor. More importantly, make sure the medication is not your only defense against drinking and develop a program of recovery to work alongside it. That way, you'll have a better chance of remaining alcohol-free once it's discontinued.

#25. Staying Stopped

most of us have tried a lot of different ways to control our drinking or drugging by the time we get to the point of quitting altogether. When we finally make the decision to stop for good, there are also many different ways we can do that. I've tried many ways of quitting myself. If you've read this book from the beginning, it's pretty obvious that I'm a chronic alcoholic who has had consistent relapses. It seemed that I could stop drinking, usually for a few months at a time, but I couldn't *stay stopped*. Maybe it was because I always wanted to find the easiest way with the least amount of effort possible. Here are some of the things I tried in those first relapse-filled years:

- Willpower
- Starting up old hobbies, including painting and drawing
- Acupuncture
- Reiki healing
- Hypnotherapy
- Herbal cleansing

- ❑ 30 day in-patient treatment program
- ❑ Relapse prevention program
- ❑ Antabuse
- ❑ Voluntarily check-in to a detox clinic
- ❑ Involuntarily check-in to a detox clinic
- ❑ Three months in a Salvation Army adult rehabilitation program
- ❑ Attempted suicide
- ❑ Psychiatric ward

As you can see from the list, there was a pretty drastic change over the years as far as the lengths that I would go to in order to quit. As I went from using willpower to attempting suicide, it was obvious that my disease, left untreated, was getting progressively worse.

I realized that I was on very shaky ground because every time I got drunk I wanted to kill myself. I didn't want to die when I was sober; it was only when I was under the influence. That's when I had the failed suicide attempt. As low as that moment was, at least it made me aware of the true scope of my problem—I knew that if I didn't stop drinking for good, it would only be a matter of time before I succeeded in ending my life.

I was out of options, and out of money, so I decided to try the one thing that I'd been avoiding for so long—a Twelve-Step program. Sure, I'd been to a few recovery meetings in the past, but I never actually listened to what those crazy people said, and I certainly never did anything they suggested. But sometimes sitting at the bottom can finally make you willing to try anything....

#26. Twelve-Step Programs

alcohol was my drug of choice, so for me the appropriate Twelve-Step program was Alcoholics Anonymous (AA). For those of us with drug addictions, there are Narcotics Anonymous (NA) and Cocaine Anonymous (CA). In addition to these, there are Twelve-Step programs for other addictions, including gambling, food, and sex (see "Recovery Resources" in the back of the book).

AA was the last stop for me. I'd been refusing to give it a chance for years, feeling as though if I went there I'd cross into new territory where I would forever be labeled an alcoholic and inducted into some kind of Bible-thumping cult. They'd find a way to change my personality and I'd be known by a different name, like Moonshine (okay, probably not that). At the very least I'd end up living in some commune, barefoot and brainwashed. Looking back on this, I guess I was a little paranoid, but I *really* wasn't excited about trying it. My choices were very limited, though; other alternatives, like in-patient treatment, were no longer an option because I was flat broke. Anyway, I'd tried them before but had never remained sober once I'd left the safety of a controlled environment.

So off I went. At my first meeting, I was told that all that was required was a desire to stop drinking (I didn't have to offer myself up as a sacrifice or anything, which seemed like good news). The travel wasn't a major challenge either, as there were meetings all over my city, as there are in most cities across the U.S., the U.K., and around the world.

If you decide to try a Twelve-Step program, but don't know where the meetings are, then rest assured that they probably won't be too hard to find. A good approach is to look under Alcoholics Anonymous, Narcotics Anonymous, or Cocaine Anonymous in your local phone book. If you have access to the Internet, www.aa.org, www.na.org, and www.ca.org have lists of meetings by city, along with phone numbers for the head offices. You can call the numbers listed locally to speak with a volunteer (confidentially), who will help you find the meeting closest to where you live. In a lot of cases they can have a volunteer meet you there, too.

Because Twelve-Step programs turned out to be such a huge topic in my sobriety, and for most of the recovering alcoholics and addicts I know, the following chapters are devoted to them: what you'll find there, how they work, and so on. For more general information, you can pick up pamphlets about the various programs either at the meeting itself or from the local chapter head office. Alternatively, most pamphlets are accessible electronically on the website of the program you are interested in.

Still, there's a lot you won't find in the pamphlets. I wish I would have known many of these things before I got started, so that's what I'll be telling you about in these remaining pages. As you read through them, keep in mind that I'm certainly not the poster child for Twelve-Step programs, and I'm not advocating that they're the *only* way to get clean and sober. However, before you dismiss them because of what you've heard from other people, or because you have preconceived ideas like I did, remember that you really have nothing to lose by trying a couple of meetings first before running for the hills.

#27. Home Groups

a home group is a Twelve-Step recovery meeting that you commit to attend on at least a weekly basis. It's suggested that you find a home group as soon as possible; it's a good way to keep grounded, and it helps you to develop a routine and a sense of familiarity. One of the most important reasons, though, is that you'll have people around who will watch your back when you stop watching it yourself.

If you attend one particular group on a regular basis, people will come to recognize and get to know you, and in the event that you stop showing up, they'll likely check up on you. Likewise, once the group is more familiar with you, the other members will be more apt to recognize a change in your behavior or attitude. Sometimes others can see a relapse coming before you can, and with any luck, they'll notice tell-tale signs and talk to you about what's going on before you get to a point of no return.

Becoming part of a home group isn't usually difficult, but we tend to make it challenging with our natural tendency to feel like outsiders. Usually it takes nothing more than showing up to a few meetings. That being said, there will be those circles where cliques evolve from groups of people that have known each other for years. For instance, I found that going to one particular group was like trying to infiltrate an Amish community, cell phones aside. In my mind, they might as well have huddled into the corner to churn butter without me. It bothered me at first, but then I realized that maybe it just wasn't a good fit for me, so I went somewhere else. If you run into a group that seems closed off, just know that most places aren't like that. Don't be put off, and remember that you can always try different settings until you find one in which you feel comfortable.

When you do find a group you are keen on, make yourself known to the person who chaired the meeting and ask how you can become a member (if they demand your firstborn child, you're probably in the wrong place). Becoming a group member is usually a matter of adding your name to the telephone list and showing up for the monthly group conscience meeting. Make sure you take a phone list for yourself, as it can be a lifesaver if you need to talk to someone about a problem, or if you are feeling like drinking or using (most groups keep their list for this exact reason).

You could also volunteer to come in early and help make the coffee, or stay after the meeting to help put away chairs. It's a great way to get to know people, and you'll be doing a service that is appreciated and needed.

#28. Look For the Similarities, Not the Differences

it's easy to look at other people and make snap judgments because of how they are dressed or the way they talk. Often, we like to do just that because it's an excuse to say, "I'm not like them so I don't belong here," or "Their problem is much worse than mine." This type of thinking puts up walls before we get a chance to know people, and it helps us continue in the illusion that we are unique.

I only had a couple of months in sobriety when I saw a girl at a meeting sitting hunched up on a chair, hiding under a baseball cap and looking like she hated the world. She was a lot younger than I was, so I figured we would have nothing in common.

We kept our distance from each other for a few weeks, until one night when we were both outside the meeting smoking a cigarette. We started talking, and it turned out she was just as nervous and intimidated as I was. As we shared our stories about how we ended up in AA, we discovered that we had a lot in common as far as our drinking histories were concerned. Suddenly, just like that, I had a friend. Since then, I've tried to be more careful about judging people based on their clothes or expressions, and my list of friends has kept growing.

You might worry that I'm about to break off into a Disney-themed life lesson—you know, this is the part where all the caterpillars dance around the beautiful butterfly to make the shape of a rainbow—but I promise you that it's just good sobriety advice. When we start to see ourselves in others, instead of apart from them, it helps us to realize that our situation is not special or different. Whether the people we meet still have their house or their spouse, and whether they have a job or not, it doesn't matter; they're still sitting in a recovery meeting because they have a substance abuse problem just like we do. We can't judge a book by its cover, because part of every person's story is similar to ours, and money or social status certainly doesn't change that or make a person more or less of an addict. The circumstances leading to another person's decline into addiction may have been different, but the problem isn't.

#29. Confidentiality

there aren't many written rules in a Twelve-Step program, but confidentiality is one of them. We are expected to respect other people's privacy, and to have them respect ours.

If you see someone you know from the outside world in a meeting, keep their attendance confidential. And if you recognize someone from a meeting when you are out in a public place, such as a supermarket, fight your first instinct to say, "Hey, don't I know you from the five o'clock Alcoholics Anonymous meeting?" In fact, it's usually best not to say anything when we see group members in public, as they might be with people who don't know about their problem.

By the same token, what you hear people talk about in the meetings needs to be kept private; it shouldn't be shared with other people outside of that room. Even gossiping and talking about what was said with other attendees should be avoided. It's bad form, and it creates the potential for things that should stay within the meeting to get out.

Gossiping and talking about other people's business is a part of life, albeit not a very nice part. Whether it's family news, work-related chatter, or a tiff between two friends, it's something we've all either observed or indulged in. But recovery meetings are especially personal, and they should stay that way. How would you feel if your most personal details were being shared inappropriately? Try to keep that in mind, and respect other people's privacy as if it were your own.

#30. Stick to Your Own Sex

When you are new to recovery meetings, stick with your own sex as far as making friends is concerned. This will help you to avoid any romantic distractions down the line.

As usual, what sounds like reasonable advice can sometimes be hard to follow. Some of us tend to make friends with the opposite sex more easily than with our own, and that might be fine outside the rooms of recovery. Inside, though, it's a risk. That's because some of these friendships might seem platonic at first, but many end up being more than that.

Like with nearly every other suggestion in this book, I had to pick things up the hard way. When I started going to meetings, most of my "friends" were men. It took some time to realize that most of them wanted my phone number for reasons other than recovery, and sometimes my intentions weren't clear either. As I mentioned earlier, not everyone is attending a meeting for the same reasons you are. There are men and women who prey on the vulnerable new faces who show up, and by sticking to your own sex, you can go a long way toward avoiding them. Once you have a bit of recovery behind you and your head is a bit clearer, you'll be able to make friends with lots of men and women, just as I did. But during those first few months, do yourself a favor and be safe rather than sorry.

If you find it hard to stay away, or if you're distracted by members of the opposite sex, try an all women or all men group; there are plenty of them around. Doing so might just keep you out of trouble—and keep you in your recovery.

#31. The Thirteenth Step

if you stick around long enough in a Twelve-Step program, chances are you'll hear about or even experience the Thirteenth Step.

The definition of this notorious 'step' is when a male or female who has usually spent a decent amount of time clean and sober (that is, enough to know better) latches onto someone who is new in recovery under the guise of wanting friendship. They introduce themselves and ask for a phone number, or to meet for coffee, seemingly offering a shoulder for the newcomer to lean on. Why is this a problem? Remember the advice: If someone of the opposite sex asks for your phone number early on, they probably want something more than a nice chat over coffee.

Unfortunately, there are some people who use the rooms of recovery as a dating pool, armed with the knowledge that the new women or men have hit rock bottom and will welcome *any* attention that is given them. After all, who better for predatory types to target than someone who has no idea how the program works? If you are in your first few months, you will need to be especially aware of this.

These "Thirteen Steppers" are pariahs and the lowest of the low. By using the tactic of feigning friendship when what they really want is sex, they aren't only messing with our emotions; they are messing with our lives. It's not unheard of for newcomers to quit going to meetings because of a bad experience. Also, being hurt and used increases the risk that they'll drink or drug again. Instead of leaving them with a bruised ego, it could kill them. If you are new in recovery and are approached by a member of the opposite sex who asks for your phone number right off the bat, politely but firmly tell them that you are there for recovery reasons, not dating reasons.

As with most things, where there's one bad apple there's bound to be a few good ones, too. And don't worry, the good ones will become easier to spot once you've got more time in recovery. A sponsor told me a story about a man with quite a few years in recovery who was attracted to a female newcomer. After looking around for some advice, he asked her if she'd consider dating him when she had gone through the Twelve Steps and reached one year of sobriety. She agreed, and after her one year sobriety birthday, they began a relationship. They celebrated their twenty-fifth wedding anniversary a few years ago.

The moral of the story is that if someone truly likes you, and is there for reasons other than finding someone to sleep with, they will wait around. Thirteen Steppers, on the other hand, are there for one thing, and one thing only, so be careful. And if you spot one, warn others before they fall for the trap.

#32. Fuck Buddies

"**F**uck Buddies" are two consenting adults who want to have sex with each other without the complications and responsibility of a relationship.

When a friend of mine mentioned that someone they knew in recovery wanted to be a "fuck buddy" with them, I nearly lost my lunch. The thought of having sex with someone you hardly know, picked from a room full of recovering alcoholics and addicts, has *bad idea* written all over it, but I guess people do it nonetheless. I asked my friend if she'd done this before, and it turned out she had and apparently it's quite common. I felt like I'd been living under a rock or something, because I hadn't a clue about it. However, after further interrogation from me, my friend admitted that it never turned out the way she thought it would, and it usually ended up with neither buddy being particularly "buddy" with the other ever again.

This might be due to the fact that alcoholics and addicts tend to have attachment issues. It's a common joke in recovery that when we go on a first date, we should expect one person to show up with moving van in tow, ready to take it to the next stage. Given that attitude, it's safe to assume that newly sober people might have a problem separating sex from love, and may ultimately want something more serious down the road, even when they initially say there are no strings attached. There's a slim chance even with "normal people" that this all-sex-no-feelings arrangement might work, but with two people who are trying to get sober, the chances of a train wreck are pretty high.

My advice is to steer clear of anyone who suggests this to you; I've heard too many *Fatal Attraction* type stories to give any other advice. You'll still have needs and feelings once your sobriety is firmly in place, so wait until you can deal with them together—or at least with a clear head.

#33. Different Strokes for Different Folks

although I've made some friends in recovery over the years, I didn't take to every person. This bothered me at first, because I thought I had to get along with everybody. Then I realized there's a difference between being polite to someone and making friends with them. We don't have to be friends with everyone, but we can at least show them some common courtesy. In other words, you can always walk away after exchanging pleasantries and no one gets offended (even if they make your skin crawl and remind you of a serial killer).

I remember a time when a man asked me for my phone number while I was still very new to recovery meetings. I really didn't want to give it to him, but I did anyway because I didn't like appearing unapproachable and unfriendly. He really gave me the creeps, so whenever he called me, I wouldn't answer the phone. Over time, I started to dread my ringtone, or worse, the thought of running into him and having to explain why I hadn't returned any of his messages. I could have avoided the whole scene if I'd just said no right off the bat when he'd asked for my number. The whole situation dragged out longer and more awkwardly than was ever necessary.

In case you've missed my point, it's this: If something like that happens to you, nip it in the bud right away. Don't hand out your number or give out personal information to people you don't want to give it to. You don't have to be Mr. or Ms. Congeniality to be in recovery, so if you have a bad feeling about someone, trust your gut and steer clear of them. Also, know your own limits. As you make friends in recovery, people might also ask to borrow money or crash on your couch for a few nights. We all want to help each other, but giving people money and letting them into your home is a whole different ball game. Wait until you've known them for at least a year before considering something like this. After that, let your conscience (and your common sense) be your guide. Remember that some people will take advantage if they can—recovery or not.

#34. Reaching Out

No matter how bad we feel our situation is, we can bet there's someone who's having it worse than we are. More often than not, we can help ourselves by being willing to help them. When we're knee deep in our own shit, though, the last thing we feel like doing is stepping in someone else's.

I remember sitting in a meeting feeling sorry for myself a week after I'd relapsed when a friend suggested that I go up and introduce myself to a newcomer who had one day sober. I scowled at my friend and asked, "What's the point? What do I know? I've only got a week myself!" He replied, "Well, you've got one week more than that poor bastard; now get your ass over there and talk to her!" He also mentioned that even though I'd relapsed, it didn't undo all that I'd learned before I drank. So I welcomed the newcomer and told her that she was in the right place. I added that I liked it so much that I'd decided to start from the beginning all over again! That small bit of humor and reassurance went a long way, and we started talking about how the program worked.

No matter where you are with your sobriety, you can look for chances to help out. It really doesn't matter if you have one week or one month; if you find yourself at a recovery meeting and see someone standing alone and uncomfortable, take a moment to introduce yourself, mention that you haven't been at this long, either, and suggest that maybe they'd like to sit with you. It's surprising how this simple gesture can make someone feel like they matter, and that they aren't invisible to the rest of the world. Besides, when we think about someone else for a moment, we stop thinking about ourselves, and that can be as powerful as anything else in recovery.

#35. Litter Mates

"**L**itter Mates" are people who start in a recovery program at the same time you do and have about the same number of weeks, months, or years sober. In early sobriety, these friendships just seem to develop without a great deal of effort because you're all in the same boat and tend to stick together. You remind one another of your new lease on life, and the last thing you want is to see one of your circle fall by the wayside.

The harsh reality, though, is that not all of us will make it and the chances that one or more of our new friends will go back out and use again is pretty high. It's just one of the hard facts of recovery, and as heartbreaking as it is, we can't take it too personally or we'll put our own progress in jeopardy.

I was very close to one of my litter mates, my first close female friend in a long time. We spent a lot of time together, and I felt like I could talk to her about anything. She even stayed at my apartment a couple of nights a week while she transitioned out of living in a recovery program halfway house. Then one day she just disappeared, and I found out from another friend that she'd used. I called and left messages, but she never called me back. She'd left all her belongings at my apartment, and she never even showed up at her job to pick up her last paycheck. She almost seemed to vanish from the earth, and afterward, I was left wondering why I hadn't seen it coming and prevented it. The same thing will likely happen to you at some point, and it's going to hurt. You'll feel abandoned, while having to deal with the stark reality that your friend is out there using, dealing with the personal hell that comes along with relapse. All you can do is hope your friend will eventually get in touch. At the same time, remember how you were when you were using. Did you usually stay in touch? I know I certainly didn't. It would have put a damper on my drinking.

It would be nice if all our litter mates would make it, but the percentages are against us. Not all these friendships will last a lifetime, and sometimes we'll get our feelings hurt by people acting strangely. Just remember that we're all just people who are trying to get well, so don't take it too personally.

For all the friends we lose, there are friends we'll keep and forge deeper connections with as we grow in recovery. I have people in my life who I have known from my early days, friends who I can count on for anything. It's a miracle that any of us even make it to the rooms of recovery; the fact that we stay there is even more amazing.

#36. What Is a Sponsor?

a sponsor is a recovering alcoholic or addict who has gone through the Twelve Steps of recovery and agrees to help you through the process. When sponsors decide to work with you, they'll take you through the steps by showing you how they did it and sharing their experience of recovery.

There's no time limit on how long it takes a person to go through the steps, but it took me a good six months to finish them. Every sponsor is different;—some might like to see you make quick progress, while others aren't going to push you to move forward at a rapid pace. There's really no right or wrong way, as long as the steps are completed thoroughly and to the best of your ability. All sponsors have their own way of going through the work (another term for the Twelve Steps), which is usually how they were shown by their sponsors. A lot of sponsors will also want to read the book of Alcoholics Anonymous or Narcotics Anonymous with you, or they may give you assignments to read certain chapters in between the times when they meet with you.

Outside of completing the steps, your sponsor will probably serve as your first line of attack against a relapse, especially early on. My first sponsor had me check in with her every day when I was very new in sobriety (under thirty days) by phone. I thought it was a pain in the ass at first, but I got used to it and making that call gave me a sense of responsibility. Some sponsors may suggest ninety meetings in ninety days, and this is a very good plan for the first three months in recovery if you can do it.

Basically their role comes down to guidance. For instance, they might introduce you to other people at the home group or meetings you attend. Or they can also answer any questions that you may have about recovery. Even if you think your questions are silly or redundant, chances are, your sponsor has heard them all before.

Think of your sponsor like you would a teacher who stays late after school to help the nervous, gawky kid because they remember what it's like to feel that way. They're there to show you the way and make sure you don't get too lost or confused. Your sponsor can't do the work for you, but they can make it clear enough so you're able to get through it.

#37. Choosing a Sponsor

It's a good idea to find a sponsor as quickly as you can. This may be someone you've seen in a meeting, have heard share, and can relate to. It's also preferable that it be a person of the same sex as you.

Having this person become your sponsor is easy. If you see someone you identify with or have a connection with, approach this person after a meeting and introduce yourself. Explain that you are new in recovery and need a sponsor, and then ask if they are taking on new people. Most will either say yes, or at least agree to be your temporary sponsor (temporary sponsorship is very common and a lot of times ends up being permanent) until you find someone else to work with. On the rare chance that they turn you down, they can probably refer you to someone else.

If you feel too awkward to approach someone and ask them personally, consider sharing in a meeting that you are looking for a sponsor. People will generally come up to you afterward if they can sponsor you, or if they know of someone who can. In addition, some groups will ask people who can sponsor to raise their hands in the meeting so newcomers will know who to ask.

When choosing a sponsor, ask yourself if you have seen your prospective sponsor at meetings. Is this person involved in the recovery community? Ask them how often they talk to *their* sponsor and the last time they went through the steps. Also ask if they're working with anyone else, as this can be good to know. If they have one or two other sponsees, that's fine, but too many could keep them very busy and limit their availability.

#38. Sponsor Misconceptions

here are a few of the misconceptions about sponsors that I had when I was a newcomer: *"A sponsor will keep you clean and sober."* It's not your sponsor's responsibility to keep you from using, which wouldn't really be possible anyway. If we are going to use, we always find a way, sponsor or no sponsor. However, if you have a sponsor and are *actively* working on the Twelve Steps, then you are arming yourself with valuable tools to fight your disease. If you feel like drinking or using, call your sponsor first. They might suggest an alternative plan of action that can turn you around.

"Sponsors can't relapse." Having a sponsor take you through the steps is one of the most vital aspects of our recovery, but it's important to remember that they are in recovery, too. They are human, just like we are, and if they are not active in a program of recovery they can relapse. You'll hear of people looking for a new sponsor because theirs "went out" (used), and that's why it's important that the person you ask to sponsor you is actively

working through a program themselves. This disease does not discriminate, and any of us can drink or use.

"A sponsor is your new best friend." While it's true that a sponsor can become a friend, don't expect to be elevated to immediate best friend status just because this person has agreed to take you through the steps; it doesn't work like that. This relationship will be a very important one, and unlike any other you have ever had before, so don't force it into becoming something it's not. Go with the flow and it will evolve as it is meant to.

#39. Sponsors vs. Therapists

therapists spend years going to school to get certified, usually have a nice office with a comfy couch, and get paid a decent salary for their troubles. Sponsors, on the other hand, have no formal training, get paid zilch, and often meet in crappy coffee shops or at their own houses.

Having been to my fair share of therapists, counselors, and psychiatrists, I can tell you that these aren't the only differences. However, this knowledge didn't stop me from treating my sponsor like a therapist the first few times we got together. She'd ask how I was doing, and I'd go off on a rant, talking about problems with my son, my job, or even my love life, expecting her to feel sorry for me and tell me everything would be okay. Much to my surprise, though, my therapist—I mean sponsor— didn't do that. She empathized with my situation, but she didn't baby me. Instead, she asked if I'd been working through the step I was on and reading what she'd suggested.

As it turned out, when I was full of self-pity and my head was off and running, I usually wasn't doing any of the things she suggested. And there's the real value of a sponsor. They might not have studied Freud for semesters on end, but they will only put up with so much of our shit before telling us we need to get off the pity pot and do some work on ourselves. Whereas a therapist gets paid to listen to our crap, no matter how boring it is or how many times we repeat it, a sponsor will tell us there is a solution to our problem. They'll tell us what to do about it, and we can either choose to follow that advice or leave it, but we don't get to whine about the situation over and over.

Keep that in mind as you meet with your sponsor. Sponsors might not have an Italian leather couch or a prescription pad, but they can offer a lot in the way of experience. In my sponsor, I found something that I couldn't get in any therapist's office— someone I could talk to and who could *really* understand what I was going through. With the professionals, I just never felt like they "got me." A sponsor, however, was a person who'd gone through the same thing and come out the other end. Talking about what bugs you is fine, but there's something invaluable about being able to spend time with someone who has already been where you are and has transformed his or her life into something better.

footnote: This shouldn't be taken to mean that you should avoid therapists, who can often be helpful in dealing with other issues that surround our addiction, including abuse, personality disorders, and other maladies.

#40. Hiring and Firing

a sponsor can fire you, and vice versa. If you have a falling out with your sponsor, get another one! This can happen. In fact, it's unusual, but not unheard of, to keep the same sponsor for the entirety of your recovered life.

There are a lot of reasons for this. It could be that your sponsor moves away from the town where you live. Family responsibilities could bring about a shift, as could a change in work schedules. And finally, sometimes people just don't mesh. Just as a series of good dates doesn't always lead to a strong long-term relationship, sometimes the initial connection isn't as clear after a while.

The first time a sponsor fired me, I was hurt and confused. After talking with other people who had more time in recovery, though, I was able to take it for what it was—a sign to move on. I decided there might be someone out there better suited to work with me. It turned out there was—I found my new sponsor the next day! The point I'm making here is that it's not that uncommon to change sponsors, for a variety of reasons, and losing yours shouldn't be cause for alarm. If you need to find another sponsor, speak up in a meeting and tell the group where you stand. Someone will step forward, or at least point you in the right direction. Once you have a new sponsor, tell them if you have started the steps or not. Your new sponsor will most likely talk with you and choose a point to start from again. It might be painful, and it's a small setback, but it's not the end of the world.

On the other hand, if you feel that you need to fire your sponsor, it doesn't have to be an awkward situation. Simply tell your sponsor politely that you appreciated working with him or her but feel it's time for you to move on. Don't make a big production of it. There's no reason to finger-point and say that your sponsor didn't do this or that; just move on amicably.

Above all, remember that so much of recovery is about learning to deal with others and ourselves. If your relationship with a sponsor dissolves, handle it like a grown-up. Don't gossip about your sponsor or the reasons for your split. Just take a look at where you are in the work, find someone new to help you, and get on with it. Not only might you work with that person again, or with someone he or she knows, you'll also be setting a good example. And since you might be a sponsor yourself someday, that's probably the best policy.

#41. A Program of Action

the Twelve-Step program is often called a program of action because we have to actually get off our asses and do some work to get results. That being said, it still took me a long time to realize that merely sitting in the meetings wasn't going to accomplish a lot. I figured that by being around all these people who were focused on their recovery, I'd absorb what they knew and put myself on the path to clean living. I was going to reach sobriety by osmosis.

For years, I'd heard successful people in recovery (meaning people with long-term sobriety) say that anyone could have what they had, if they would just do the work—but I didn't know what the work was. It turns out that they meant working on the Twelve Steps. I had the equation half right. I wanted what they had; I just didn't want to do anything to get it. Finally, after another relapse, I decided to get a sponsor and do the Twelve Steps. I still didn't see what the fuss was about. I just *knew* they wouldn't do anything for me, and that I'd fall off the wagon again in a few months. Still, I was tired of hearing everyone tell me to do the work and I wanted them off my back, so I announced to my friends that I would complete the steps. After my grand proclamation, I expected them to say, "Great news!" or at least, "Well done!" Their actual response, however, was a bit more tepid: "It's about fucking time."

It's not that I was alone. While actually *doing* the Steps may sound like an obvious part of the process, you'd be surprised at how many people attend recovery meetings but have not completed them. They're still stuck in that in-between zone like I was—not drinking or using, but not really happy, either. That's because the meetings alone might keep us sober for a while, but eventually we need more than that, and the steps offer a solution. Even if you're like I was and think the program won't work for you, do yourself a favor and try. I can almost promise you'll learn just what I did: that by not drinking or using we might be able to survive, but with recovery, we can live.

#42. A Design for Living

to the uninitiated, *The Twelve Steps of Recovery* can sound a lot like *The Twelve Things to Get at the Grocery Store*, or *The Twelve Things to Do Today*—a list of loosely assorted things to scratch off or move through. When I began the work, however, I learned that this isn't the case. There's reasoning behind the number of steps, as well as their placement, that makes them so effective. In other words, it matters that there are a dozen of them, and they work when they are done in their entirety and in the order in which they're written.*

Probably the best advice I could pass on is this: *Concentrate on the step you are on and don't worry about the next one.* Each one is just as important as the one before and after it.

I could also add that Step One, *admitting that we're powerless over our addiction and that our lives have become unmanageable,* was very difficult for me, as it is for many people. That's because even though I knew deep down that I had a problem with alcohol, I really had a hard time admitting it to myself. Eventually, after experiencing relapse upon relapse, and losing everything over and over again, I reached a point where I was willing to admit that I was indeed an alcoholic, that I was powerless over alcohol, and that my life was way beyond unmanageable. I finally had my first step, which is the key to all the others.

As you progress through the rest of the steps, remember that a recovery program is also called a "design for living" because as each step unfolds we come to understand more about ourselves and a different way to live. Moreover, the steps give us a way to rebuild our lives by cleaning up the past. In doing so, we are shown how to live without guilt, remorse, and fear.

See the book of Alcoholics Anonymous or Narcotics Anonymous for a list of the Twelve-Steps.

#43. What is a Higher Power?

One of my biggest reasons for staying away from Twelve-Step programs had always been the God factor. I don't have strong religious convictions, but I had long ago formed an impression of a being that had long since stopped giving a shit about me and thought I was basically just taking up space on the planet.

Consequently, when I walked into the rooms of recovery, my stomach lurched the moment I saw the references to God and heard talk of the "fellowship." I felt like I'd turn into a pillar of salt at any given moment, or at least be singled out and refused entry because of the obvious dirt on my soul. I was somewhat surprised when that didn't happen, and what's more, I found out that there were people in these meetings who seemed to feel the same way I did. The uneasiness I felt quickly returned, though, when I started working the Twelve Steps and was told that for Steps Two and Three, I would need to believe in a power greater than myself that could restore me to sanity. I would have to turn my will and my life over to the care of God as I understood Him.

That was going to be a problem, because I didn't understand God at all. In fact, I had quite a few beefs with Him/Her/It, and I tended to obsess about them on a regular basis. I didn't understand, for instance, why there were starving, homeless people in one part of the world, while people with more money than sense are living in another, squandering it on gold-plated Mercedes, two or three homes, and diamond pet collars. Needless to say, I wasn't sold on the idea of turning my will over to something I didn't understand at all.

Thankfully, I had a very patient and knowledgeable sponsor who explained that it wasn't a matter of understanding God; it was about a God of my understanding, which was completely different. I didn't even need to call it God; it could be called a Higher Power, the Great Pumpkin, Rat-Bastard, or basically anything I wanted, just as long as it was something I could envisage being bigger and more powerful than myself, because it was my interpretation.

Once I realized what the third step actually meant, I found that I could get on board with my own idea of a Higher Power, and I set about conjuring up an image of one.

It took me a while, but I was able to finally decide what my concept of a Higher Power was. Not long after, I met with my sponsor and explained my conception of it: My God had a sense of humor, was non-judgmental, made sure there were no super-rich people or really poor people, loved me unconditionally, wasn't bothered by my lack of sensitivity to religious idols, and was very approachable, patient, and certainly not holier-than-thou. And as one last thing, He happened to look and behave a lot like the God portrayed by the actor Morgan Freeman in the movie *Bruce Almighty*. He was definitely more powerful than me, but not in an intimidating way. In fact, he had more of an unassuming manner, and was not opposed to mopping the floors now and again or changing a light bulb. As I said before, my sponsor was very patient, and so Morgan Freeman it was.

Lest you should think mine is the only Higher Power with an offbeat personality or celebrity status, let me mention that I've even heard someone say Mickey Mouse was theirs (although I didn't get that one—he's really tiny!). The point is, it is up to you to decide. Just because many people use a certain concept of God as a Higher Power, that doesn't mean you have to follow suit. That's the beauty of a Twelve-Step program; we are free to choose a Higher Power of *our understanding*.* It doesn't really matter what we name it, or how we think of it, so long as it's there.

As addicts and alcoholics, we tend to be selfish and self-centered. This isn't meant as an insult; it's the very nature of our disease. If we can believe there is something out there more powerful than ourselves, then we can begin to look outside of our own egos and start to lose the need to be in control. And very often, that cuts to the heart of our need to drink or use. Whatever point we are at in recovery, but especially early on, there's no denying we can use all the help we can get—that's what your Higher Power is all about.

---

* In case you're interested, entire books have been written on this subject, but rather than walk into a philosophical minefield, I just want to keep it simple and invite you to your own research and conclusions.

#44. The Atheist and Agnostic

It's easy to be put off Twelve-Step programs by the emphasis on finding a Higher Power and all the talk of God. For me, it wasn't so much of a problem that I couldn't get past it. If you're a true atheist or agnostic, though, you might not want to engage in those discussions. Luckily, there are alternatives (see the end of this chapter). There are new recovery programs springing up, designed by people just like you who would rather keep religion and recovery in separate jars.

The only obstacle or difference that I would point out in one of these programs is their relative rarity. There aren't many of them around yet, and they don't have a lot of meetings in many cities. I'm hopeful that this will change over time, as these programs seem to be a growing trend. I can't say a lot about them personally. Having looked into the different options available to me, I was aware of some of these organizations, but there were none in my vicinity and I wanted to physically be around other people in recovery. If you are in a similar situation and the only option seems to be a Twelve-Step group or nothing, then maybe there is a way that you can make the program work with the beliefs that you have.

A Higher Power is the belief that there is something out there more powerful than ourselves. Some people I've met in recovery who were atheist or agnostic were able to use their home group or the actual rooms of recovery themselves as a Higher Power. In fact, I've heard some use the acronym Group of Drunks (G.O.D.) as a way of getting this message across. All they needed was the willingness to believe that there's something out there bigger and more powerful than they are, and a group of people together as a whole is definitely a greater force than one person. This solution has worked for a lot of people, and it might be an answer that works for you—at least until you have (or start) a suitable group in your area.

Along the same lines, I would ask, does it really matter how we get clean and sober, as long as we get there? Most of us are at a point where we're willing to try anything to stop living the way we have been. In my years of recovery, I've heard a number of religious sentiments that I didn't agree with, but none of them has interfered with my own sobriety. Not every person, or idea, makes sense to everybody, but each of us has our own path to walk.

Alternative programs: Other non-religious and non-spiritual programs are Agnostic AA; Rational Recovery; Self-Management and Recovery Training: SMART; Women for Sobriety; Men for Sobriety; and Secular Organizations for Sobriety: also known as "Save Our Selves," or SOS. A list of contact information for these organizations can be found in the back of this book with the suggested reading materials.

#45. 'Not So Great' Expectations

any good recovery program is as much a journey of self-discovery as it is a treatment for an addiction. Very often, by taking the time to reflect on our own habits and behaviors, we discover unhealthy thoughts or patterns that we've had for a long time.

One of the underlying problems we tend to have is expectations. An expectation is a hope, belief, want, or desire that is typically linked to a person or event. In other words, alcoholics and addicts are bogged down with expectations because we regularly expect people to do what we want, or expect things to go our way. We continually set ourselves up for disappointment because we think people are our puppets to do with as we please, pulling their strings to get them to act in a way we deem appropriate. The problem with this is that other people are fallible, as are we, and so we end up disappointed. And where there is disappointment or hurt, there will ultimately be resentment (which I'll cover in the next chapter).

In fact, you might hear people in recovery say that an expectation is a resentment waiting to happen, which turns out be true. We can't make people jump through the hoops we want. We only need to look at ourselves for proof; have we ever been able to get ourselves to do what we want?

Even once we acknowledge the trouble with expectations, trying to control people is a very hard habit to break. For example, my sister and her family recently came to visit me from England and I wanted everything to be perfect. Since I live in Colorado, this isn't a quick or easy trip. They were understandably exhausted, so when we picked them up at the airport in the evening, we took them straight to their hotel. The first thing I did in the morning, though, was call my sister's hotel room. Rather than ask if she'd managed to get some sleep after her twenty-hour journey, I immediately blurted out, "Did you look at the Rocky Mountains yet?" She replied, of course, that they hadn't, because they'd not been awake very long. I almost screamed at her, "What? You've come all this way and haven't even looked out your window to see the mountains? Go and look right now while I'm on the phone!" (You'd think I had actually arranged to have them put out there especially for her). It was ridiculous, and as soon as I said it, I thought, *What the hell am I doing? Here I am trying to make her look out of her window at the mountains so she'll think about what a great job I did getting her a hotel with this spectacular view.* I was already expecting her to behave and react in a certain way, and when she didn't, I got agitated.

I actually shared this incident in a recovery meeting that both my sister and I went to while she was visiting. We had a good laugh about it, and so did everyone else. They could relate, because this is what alcoholics and addicts do—we expect things to go a certain way, and for people to behave and react the way we want. Then if our expectations are not met, we get resentful.

As people in recovery, we need to be mindful of our motives on a daily basis. Our lives will become easier to manage; by expecting less, we will resent less. Thankfully, I was able to recognize this old behavior with my sister and nip it in the bud, and we were able to relax and enjoy the time we had together (in the spectacular, awe-inspiring, jaw-dropping Rocky Mountains).

#46. Resentment

Someone once said to me that having resentment was like drinking a bottle of poison and expecting someone else to die from it. That stuck with me because it summed up the futility of harboring resentment and just how dangerous it can be. Basically, resentment is a feeling of anger or bitterness, usually directed toward another person or persons, living or dead. It's not that uncommon, though, to harbor resentment toward other entities, such as employers, organizations, government, police, and religious institutions—pretty much anything! As humans, we all have resentments; the reason I'm mentioning them here has to do with the way normal people deal with them versus the way alcoholics and addicts deal with them.

If someone offends a normal person, that person might address the issue right away, or just let it go without giving it a second thought (a concept completely foreign to alcoholics and addicts). For the addicted mind, however, the offense becomes a preoccupation no matter how large or small it is. As if that weren't unhealthy enough, these preoccupations can easily lead to drinking or using.

When I first came into recovery, I had no idea about resentments, and how alcoholics and addicts are ruled by them. Anger and disappointment were so much a part of me, a seething mass of bitterness and frustration, that I didn't give these feelings a second thought until my sponsor started talking about the subject.

As we talked about these feelings, it became apparent that I was keeping dozens and hundreds of them, holding on to them and repeating them in my mind. My sponsor went on to explain that this isn't unusual; alcoholics and addicts are notoriously bad forgetters. We hang on to every slight or unkind word, giving them more and more power over us until every perceived injustice feels overwhelming, no matter how small or large it actually is.

So, how do we deal with our past and all of our hurts and anger? By working through a Twelve-Step program, since one of the steps is specifically designed to acknowledge and address the resentments we have, from the very old to the brand new. What's more, it involves a tried and tested way to deal with old wounds in a manner specifically designed for alcoholic and addicts.

Be aware that even with a program in place, this will take some time and effort. Part of the process involves recognizing our feelings for what they are and seeing if we have a part in the resentment. It can be tough to accomplish, but the freedom we get to feel afterward is indescribable.

As I was discussing these issues with my sponsor, she asked if I knew that resentments are known as the number one killer of alcoholics and addicts. I didn't see how that made sense; how could being angry with someone kill me? She went on to explain that if we do not deal with anger and hurt, we drive ourselves crazy thinking about it until we do what we always do to quiet our minds—we pick up and use alcohol or drugs. Resentments can kill because for some of us, the next time we use might very well be the last time.

I chose to follow a Twelve-Step program because it was my last resort. While my reasons weren't ideal, it was by far the best decision I could have made at that time in my life. Instead of spending a ton of money and countless hours with a therapist, I was shown a way to lose my emotional baggage that was constructive, effective, and free of charge. The relief I felt when I finally let go of so much is beyond words. More importantly, when new resentments arise (which is a daily occurrence), I now have a way to address them without letting them run free through my mind.

Dealing with these is paramount because they affect our mental health, and ultimately our physical health, since we use drugs or alcohol to mask the pain.

Facing our resentments is one of *the most important* components to continued sobriety. Thankfully, the process for working with them is available to all of us through the Twelve-Step program if we are just willing to do a little work.

#47. Ego and Fear

Part of the work involved in addressing my resentments was writing them all down, along with the feelings I associated with them.

One example was a resentment against a former friend of mine, who I felt was two-faced and untrustworthy because of the way she had treated me. She had said some things behind my back, which had left me angry and hurt. My sponsor listened while I explained the situation, then told me that the resentment was less a result of my friend's behavior than a result of my ego. I was skeptical, but I decided to listen anyway.

Before too long, I began to see what my sponsor meant. While I thought I was angry over some things this person had said after I'd relapsed, the real reason for my fury was that she had rejected me as a friend. I hated feeling like I was not good enough for someone's friendship, and that's what stung so deeply.

By looking at this example with another person (my sponsor), I was able to identify one of my character defects: jealousy, and the underlying fear of rejection. Sure, I disguised the fear with anger, but beneath that anger was definitely fear. A light seemed to come on when I realized this. As I went through the remainder of my resentments, I could see how ego and fear were intertwined with all of them.

That probably doesn't sound like great news, but you can't fix what you can't see, and I never would have been able to recognize and face up to these challenges on my own and without the help of my sponsor. It's not easy to visit the darker corners of our selves. Sometimes big fears are involved, along with other emotions we'd rather not feel, much less see. Only by dealing with them, however, can we tear ourselves free of their grip. Without self-knowledge, we're doomed to continue acting out the same scripts and scenes, each with their own sad endings. By moving through the steps and facing our demons, however, we find a way to remove them and a chance at a new beginning.

#48. Making Amends

if we are to successfully continue in recovery, it's imperative that we make amends with the people in our lives who we have hurt, angered, used, abused, harmed, and offended (you get the idea). This might take more courage and effort than you think. Contrary to popular belief, making amends is not simply saying we are sorry; it is about being willing to make restitution for what we have done.

It can be overwhelming to think of our past and the things we've done, under the influence or not. (That's why it is strongly recommended that you do this with a sponsor as part of a Twelve-Step program.) Many of us stopped at nothing to get our drug of choice, and once we got our fix, we continued to lie and cheat, blazing our way through people's lives without giving them a second thought. That's why most alcoholics and addicts are riddled with guilt, of which they must free themselves if they're to remain sober and happy. Making amends is not only the right thing to do for our own sake, but because in doing so, the people we have hurt can heal and move forward. And if they can, so can we.

I used to think that just being clean and sober was enough to make things right. Surely the people I'd hurt could see that I was different now—shouldn't that make everything okay? I sincerely thought I was so special that people would forgive me all my indiscretions merely because I'd stopped using. Naturally, I was wrong. Keeping sober was not going to rid me of the consequences of my addiction.

As part of the amends process, we must make a list of the people we have harmed and are willing to make amends to, unless the admission will cause that person more harm than if we didn't make amends at all. In other words, we set out to right the wrongs that we can.

There are different kinds of amends. First, there are the ones we make to loved ones, friends, co-workers, and acquaintances. There are also living and financial amends, as well as the amends we make to those who have passed away and are no longer with us.

As I mentioned earlier, this undertaking should be done under the guidance of a sponsor. My sponsor went over the basic idea with me a few times, helped me compile a list, and then gave me some guidelines on how to carry it through. The most important guideline was to trust in my Higher Power to get me through the really difficult ones.

There are also the living amends. These are the small ones that we need to keep making every day, for those people we can't adequately set right with any one action. I asked my ex-husband on a few occasions if I could speak with him concerning amends (having explained the process to him before), but I could tell he wasn't comfortable with it, so I didn't push the issue. Instead, I just continued to do what I had been doing already, continuing to be present, reliable, honest, and a good mother to our son. This is an example of a living amend. Usually, these are the kind we make to our families, spouses, and children. We can't ever change the past; all we can do is live each day as best we can.

We must keep in mind that this process is about the harm that we have inflicted, not about pointing fingers at other people for things *they* may have done. Nothing will ruin an amends more than saying at the end of it, "Okay, now it's your turn!" Your amend is about what you did, say what you need to say and leave it at that.

Essentially, we are cleaning up our past. Not only is this the right thing to do, it also indicates a level of sincerity and integrity on our part that might have been lacking in the past. Be careful, though, of expectations of tearful reunions; once we have done our part, we must let it be. There are times when you'll never get that storybook ending. In making my amends, I wrote a letter to a woman who had been my best friend for several years. In the body, I explained the process I'd been working through and expressed my regret at having damaged our relationship with my drinking. Unfortunately, I never heard back from her. And even though it hurt to know she'd probably decided against having any more contact with me, I had to understand her point of view. We have all hurt people immeasurably and have to respect their privacy. We do this by not pursuing them after we've made the initial contact. We just have to trust that if they want to get in touch with us, they will. Beyond that, it's out of our hands and in that of our Higher Power's. Besides, there are so many unseen miracles that could happen months or years down the line that you can do the right thing without ever giving up that last bit of hope.

Another word of advice: Make *all* of your amends. Don't put them off until later, and try not to think of the "what ifs." Just deal with them as best you can, and then live in the present. We don't have to like who we were, but we are not the same people anymore, and once we face up to the past, we're free to live in a better present.

#49. Recovery Rut

another acronym you will hear in recovery is *R.I.D.*, which is **R**estless, **I**rritable, and **D**iscontent. Basically, these amount to the feelings that surface when we're caught in a rut in our recovery, doing the same things (with the same people) day in and day out.

Fortunately, while R.I.D. might seem like a heavy acronym, it's a pretty easy problem to fix. Humans thrive on variety and surprise, so recognize that your mind is going to want a break from its usual diet from time to time.

One good way to keep things fresh is by checking out a different group or meeting. Just because you might have chosen a home group, that doesn't have to be the only group you attend. Besides the fact that home groups have the same people who invariably share every time, there are so many different groups to choose from that it would be silly to never check out any others. Most cities have women-only groups, men-only groups, and gay and lesbian groups. Get into the habit of trying one different meeting every week or two. The fact that it's convenient to go to the meeting down the street doesn't mean that it's the best meeting for you. Even if your normal meeting does turn out to be the best one, at least you'll have looked at things from a different perspective, with its own voices and faces, for just a little while.

Obviously, I'm partial to writing. Even if you don't plan on ever finishing a book, though, you might give it a try. Writing in a daily journal can be cathartic and a great way of opening up and venting. All you need is a few moments to put down your thoughts about the day that's passed. It doesn't matter if it was great, terrible, or something in-between. Simply note your thoughts and impressions as they come to you—you might be surprised at what comes out. Alternately, if you're still feeling a bit gloomy, jot down something that you are grateful for. Sometimes, it may be only one thing, "being clean and sober." If that's all you can manage to write, then write that. You might find you have more to say tomorrow. If nothing else, you'll be left with something you can come back to later for reflection. My journal from the first year has me ranting one day and eternally grateful the next, but it gave me a lot of insight when I looked at it months down the line and saw how bat-shit crazy I really was (and still am).

Another way to get out of your own head and to cure irritability is to help others, and this is the final (and some would say most important) piece of a Twelve-Step program. Sometimes it may feel like the last thing in the world that you want to do, but by helping others, we invariably help ourselves. There are so many people in recovery meetings, detox meetings, treatment centers, halfway houses, and prisons who are struggling with the same disease that you are. By sharing your story, you might spark a light of change in someone else's life. And there's not really anything, in your development in recovery or in life, as fulfilling as that.

Helping others doesn't need to be restricted to other people in recovery, either. It can be as simple as taking the time to listen, instead of waiting for another person to stop talking so you can have your say. Showing other people the simple courtesy of giving your uninterrupted attention to what they have to say will speak volumes about you. The small things, no matter how trivial, add up. And they *do* matter. Try saying good morning to your neighbor instead of grunting and rushing off, put the grocery cart back when you are done with it, open the door for someone, or just let someone in front of you in traffic (that one took me a while). These might seem like inconsequential actions, but they help us remember to stop rushing through our lives, be present in the moment, and appreciate the small things that make up our day.

As we spend more time in recovery, we tend to forget how bad it used to be. As a result, we can become discontented even when things are a hundred times better than they ever were. Don't forget where you came from, but don't dwell on it either. That's why milestones are important; they let us celebrate our achievements, while at the same time allowing us to take a quick glimpse in the rearview mirror. So acknowledge it when you put some chunk of sobriety behind you. It doesn't matter if it's one month or six, or whether you're in a Twelve-Step program or not; the occasion is important. Do something nice for yourself: Buy a book, get your hair done, or go out to dinner with your loved ones. You have been given a second chance at life, so bloody well get out there and start living it!

#50. Progress, Not Perfection

I used to think "sober and happy" was an oxymoron. After my experiences as a dry drunk I absolutely, without a doubt, considered it impossible to be both at the same time. As far as I was concerned, I'd be destined to forever obsess about alcohol and never have any fun. Thankfully, I was wrong.

While each day doesn't start out like a Disney movie, it doesn't end like a horror movie either (which was usually the case when I was using). I know that finding inner peace is not impossible if I'm willing to follow directions and do some work. It may be difficult at times, but it's worth it in the long-run.

The best part is, I've learned we don't have to be perfect. We don't have to become Twelve-Step gurus, holding all the answers and quoting verbatim from recovery books. We can take ideas for what they are, without accepting everything that comes in or dismissing everything that makes us uncomfortable. We don't have to like everyone and agree with all that's said. In short, we're free to be people, warts and all, progressing toward a better ideal but living our lives here in the real world.

I didn't think the steps would work for me, *but* I was willing to try them anyway. I took a leap of faith. And much to my surprise, I didn't become a brainwashed member of a cult. Instead, as I started working on myself, I realized that I was feeling better about my recovery and thinking less and less about using. Eventually, working my way through the Twelve Steps, my obsession with alcohol was lifted— something I never thought I'd be able to say honestly in a million years. The funny thing is, I can't pinpoint the day it happened; it was more of a gradual shift. I was so involved with my new life and what that entailed—the recovery meetings, the step work, and spending time with my son—that one day I just realized I hadn't thought about alcohol once that day, and I guess that's the proof in the pudding. Here I was, this hopeless, resentful, relapsing chronic alcoholic, and then suddenly alcohol didn't own me anymore. That's my miracle.

Over time, as our minds, bodies, and spirits begin to heal, we can learn to better monitor ourselves. Not every thought has to last for hours; not every impulse has to be followed to its end. Better yet, we can learn to laugh at ourselves and understand our crazier thoughts for what they are: thoughts, not realities.

This is a lifelong disease. There is no cure, but there is treatment for those of us who want it. This journey we are on is truly about making progress, not achieving perfection. We don't suddenly turn into saints because we put our drug of choice down. We are works in progress. There will be bad days, but there will be great days, too.

Along the way, your perception of what being happy means might change. Mine certainly did, evolving into something completely different than what it had been when I started. Today, it's *peace of mind* that makes me happy, when my head is still, no hamsters and no static, free from guilt, resentment, and a constant barrage of irrational thoughts and fears. I used to live with these things every day; not having them anymore is truly amazing. It's not always smooth sailing, but when I'm pissed off at the world, I figure out why and what my part in it is, and then I fix it.

For me, this was made possible by having a program of recovery in place, including the willingness to listen to the suggestions of others, do the work on the steps, go to recovery meetings, have a sponsor, and make sober friends. Most importantly, I fostered a spiritual relationship with a Higher Power and turned my will over to it on a daily basis. As I broke the chains of my addiction, I learned a very important lesson: our freedom comes with a very small price. As recovering alcoholics and addicts, it's our mission and responsibility to help other people who are suffering to find *their* way, too, just as others have helped us. Our stories can be invaluable, as they might just bring a glimmer of hope to those who are now standing where we once stood.

We might have this disease until the day we die, but we can choose to die *with* it, not *from* it. In the meantime, we owe it to ourselves to live each day to the fullest and remember never to let the bastards grind us down.

Recovery Resources

This list was put together specifically with alcoholics and addicts in mind, and it lists the programs relative to alcoholism and drug addiction. This is not a full and complete list of all the Twelve-Step programs available, but only the programs that pertain to substance abuse:

Twelve-Step Programs:
(In alphabetical order, not in order of preference)

Agnostic AA (USA & France)	www.agnosticaanyc.org
Al-Anon and Alateen (USA)	www.al-anon.alateen.org
Al-Anon and Alateen (UK & Eire)	www.al-anonuk.org.uk
Alcoholics Anonymous (USA)	www.alcoholics-anonymous.org
Alcoholics Anonymous (UK)	www.alcoholics-anonymous.org.uk
Cocaine Anonymous (USA	www.ca.org
Cocaine Anonymous (UK)	www.cauk.org.uk
Crystal Meth Anonymous (USA)	www.crystalmeth.org
Dual Recovery Anonymous (USA)	www.draonline.org
Narcotics Anonymous (USA)	www.na.org

Other Recovery Programs (Not Twelve-Step Progams):
(In alphabetical order, not in order of preference)

LifeRing	www.unhooked.com
Rational Recovery (USA)	www.rational.org
SMART Recovery (USA)	www.smartrecovery.org
SMART Recovery (UK)	www.smartrecovery.co.uk
SOS, "Save Our Selves"	www.secularsobriety.org
Women for Sobriety (USA)	www.womenforsobriety.org

Suggested Reading

This list is based on books that are recommended by and for people in recovery. They are available in most major book stores and online book stores.

Alcoholics Anonymous Big Book, 4th Edition
By AA Services, Publisher: Alcoholics Anonymous World Services, Inc.; Forth edition (2002)

Twelve Steps and Twelve Traditions
By AA Services, Publisher: Hazelden (2002)

Narcotics Anonymous
By Narcotics Anonymous, Publisher: Hazelden Publishing & Educational Services; Fifth edition

Hope, Faith and Courage: Stories from the Fellowship of Cocaine Anonymous
Publisher: Cocaine Anonymous World Services

How Al-Anon Works for Families & Friends of Alcoholics
By Al-Anon Family Group Head, Inc., Publisher: Al-Anon Family Group Headquarters, Inc.

Came to Believe
By AA Services, Publisher: Hazelden (2002)

Keep It Simple: Daily Meditations For Twelve-Step Beginnings And Renewal
By Anonymous, Publisher: Hazelden (1996)

The Dark Night of Recovery: Conversations from the Bottom of the Bottle
By Edward Bear, Publisher: HCI (1999)

The Tao of Pooh
By Benjamin Hoff, Publisher: Penguin (Non-Classics); First edition (1983)

Adult Children of Alcoholics
By Janet G. Woititz, Publisher: HCI; Expanded edition (1990)

Emotional Sobriety: The Next Frontier: Selected Stories from the AA Grapevine
By AA Grapevine, Inc., Publisher: AA Grapevine Inc. (2006)

The Dual Disorders Recovery Book
By Anonymous, Publisher: Hazelden; First edition (1993)

Tweak: Growing Up on Methamphetamines
By Nic Sheff, Publisher: Ginee Seo Books (2008)

Addict In The Family: Stories of Loss, Hope, and Recovery
By Beverly Conyers, Publisher: Hazelden; First edition (2003)

The Steps We Took
By Joe McQ., Publisher: August House (1990)

Drop The Rock: Removing Character Defects, Steps Six and Seven, Second Edition
By Bill P., Todd W., Sara S., Publisher: Hazelden;
Second edition (March 1, 2005)

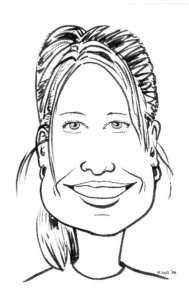

Georgia W. is a part-time writer and full-time recovering alcoholic. She was born near Manchester, England and now lives in Denver, Colorado with her very significant other and her son (and the occasional hamster). If you would like to contact Georgia, please visit www.early-recovery.com or email: georgia@early-recovery.com.